Thomas Berthelet

Royal Printer and
Bookbinder to Henry VIII.
King of England

Cyril Davenport

Alpha Editions

This edition published in 2023

ISBN : 9789357941792

Design and Setting By
Alpha Editions
www.alphaedis.com
Email - info@alphaedis.com

Contents

CHAPTER I.

ENGLISH BOOKBINDING UP TO THE TIME OF HENRY VIII.

Such English bookbindings of an early date as still exist are, as a rule, bound in dark brown goatskin or brown sheepskin. The earliest notices about bookbindings are to be found in some of the wardrobe accounts of Edward IV., but of the many bindings which were made for that king, the only remaining sign now left is a loose cover in the library of Westminster Abbey; it is ornamented with a panel stamp bearing the king's arms, with supporters.

In Mediæval times, books, mostly religious, were generally written, copied, illuminated, and bound in the monasteries themselves, and were frequently of large size. After the date at which printing was introduced into Europe, about the middle of the fifteenth century, books became commoner, and very soon, as a general rule, smaller, the printer, binder, and publisher usually combining in his own person the functions hitherto performed by separate artists and artificers,—the illuminators, scribes, silversmiths, goldsmiths, jewellers, enamellers, and workers in leather, wood, or ivory. In short, the art of producing books became in every way a less ornamental and a commoner one.

It is disappointing that no single specimen of the rich Mediæval style of bookbinding exists of English workmanship. Such bindings were undoubtedly made here, and numerous drawings of them are to be seen in contemporary manuscript. It is certain that the intrinsic value of these covers attracted the attention of some of our sovereigns, especially the early Tudors, and whenever they were of any value at all, the crucible accounts for their disappearance. Luckily the manuscripts themselves, now infinitely more valuable than the gold and silver which formerly covered them, have in innumerable instances been carefully preserved unhurt. But it is some comfort to know that much beautiful work of the kind we have so unfortunately lost here can be seen and studied in Dublin, at the Royal Irish Academy and other institutions. In that city are to be seen noble specimens of the old book shrines, or covers, which protected the valuable manuscripts, illuminated sometimes by the ancient Irish scribes in such richness that they have never been excelled in beauty. These covers are in all probability nearly the same as the English ones were; they bear ornamentation of a similar Gothic character, nearly analogous to the Anglo-Saxon styles, and the jewels are cut and set in the same way as is found in old English jewellers' work. The "cumdach," or cover, of Molaise's Gospels, that of the Stowe missal and

"Dimma's book," are all beautiful examples. The Irish jewellers were justly celebrated workmen; they migrated largely to the Continent, and traces of their skill often show on Byzantine bindings made from about the ninth to the eleventh centuries. The older part of the magnificent cover of the Gospels of Lindau is Irish work. This was shown in 1891 at the Burlington Fine Art Club, and until lately was the property of the Earl of Ashburnham. It is one of the most gorgeous bookbindings in existence.

In some Eastern countries bordering on Europe, especially the north of Africa and parts of Asia, books were bound in leather and ornamented with gold at a very early date. Signs of such work are found on bindings of the twelfth century onwards, but it is always rare, and only sparingly used. The manner of working the gold differs considerably from the way it is treated now. Persian, Arabian, and Egyptian work of this sort is of great interest, and well deserves more attention and examination than it has yet received. It even seems that some kind of gilding on books was practised in England as early as 1480, as appears from one of the accounts of Piers Courteys, keeper of the King's Great Wardrobe in the City of London; but there is not enough information given to enable us to say what sort of gilding this was, neither do the existing specimens throw any definite light on this particular point.

The account in which this reference to gilding on books occurs is one of the entries referring to the Privy Purse Expenses of Elizabeth of York, daughter of Edward IV., and afterwards wife to Henry VII.; the words are as follows:—

"Piers Bauduyn stacioner for bynding gilding and dressing of a booke called *Titus Livius* XX^s; for binding gilding and dressing of a booke of *The Holy Trinite* XVj^s; for binding gilding and dressing of a booke called *The Bible* XVj^s; for binding gilding and dressing of a booke called *Le Gouvernment* of Kings and Princes XVj; ... and for binding and gilding and dressing of a booke called The Bible Historial XX^s."

It is, I think, probable that these bindings were ornamented with panel stamps, which were simply gilded all over, and that the process referred to was not that which is now generally understood as gold-tooling.

During the Middle Ages Venice was the most important European centre of trade with Eastern countries, and so it naturally comes about that the first European gold-tooling on leather comes from that great art centre, and occurs in Italian bindings of the fifteenth century. Not only does gold-tooling first appear in Venetian work, but there also it reached its highest development, several of the early bindings tooled in gold on dark leathers being quite unsurpassed for delicacy and originality of design, as well as for beauty of workmanship. In several of these bindings the direct inspiration that has been afforded by the study of Oriental originals is very apparent.

Innumerable also are the methods the Italian artists followed with regard to their management of gold leaf, or gold foil; sometimes a whole design is picked out with minute gold dots, sometimes backgrounds are flatly gilded all over, leaving the design on the leather, and sometimes the method of working closely resembles that followed at the present day. The early Venetian bookbinders, as well as some of the Oriental gilders, knew some way of gilding a line drawn on leather by means of a style. This is a difficult thing to do, but effective in competent hands; and if it could be done with any degree of safety, such a process would now open up an entirely new field for decorative bookbinders, who are at present much bound down by the limitations forced upon them in consequence of chiefly using set stamps specially cut for each curve and bend and detail. Of course such lines are easy to execute in blind, but it is when the gilding begins that the difficulties increase. The essential point in gold-tooling on leather, as we know it, consists in the fixation of gold leaf by means of albumen. The design is marked in blind on leather and painted over with glair of egg, the gold leaf then being carefully laid over it; the marks of the blind-tooling show clearly through the gold, and each of these impressions is steadily reimpressed with the same tools in the same places over the gold. The tools are heated to a point just sufficient to harden the albumen without burning the leather. If necessary, this process can be repeated again and again, until in the finest specimens of such work the gold looks as if wires of the solid burnished metal were actually inlaid on the leather. The albumen protected by the gold

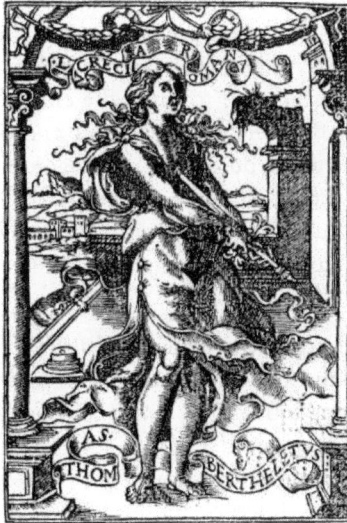

PLATE III.

BERTHELET'S DEVICE OF LUCRETIA STABBING HERSELF.

makes such a strong surface that frequently the gilded letters, or designs, which were of course originally in *intaglio*, are found in relief, the explanation being that the surrounding leather, being unprotected, has worn or powdered away all around. The use of albumen is, however, not entirely without a drawback, as it is a favourite food for some small grub, so that sometimes, instead of a beautiful gilded line, there is only a small trench following the same track, all the gold and all the albumen having been eaten away, leaving the design as it was, but in a different colour.

As a matter of fact, the earliest English binding now existing on which gold occurs is in the Bodlein Library at Oxford, but it would hardly come under the heading of gold-tooling. It is on a manuscript written by Robert Witinton about 1516, and was given by him to Cardinal Wolsey. The binding is in brown sheepskin, and is decorated with block impressions from panel stamps, three on each side, the centre one representing St. George and the dragon, and the side ones bearing the Tudor emblems, portcullis, pomegranate, and double rose. These stamps are well and boldly cut, and the impressions are gilded, but I think it would be difficult to say positively whether they were simply overlaid with gold leaf after being made on the leather, or whether the gold was fixed by the operation of stamping. I rather expect the latter method was used; but the volume is a very curious and interesting one even if such is not the case, and to some extent may explain the gilding mentioned in Piers Courteys's account.

In England during the fifteenth century the printing, binding, and publishing of printed books generally vested in the same individual, but by degrees these processes became specialized, and towards the end of the sixteenth century they were carried out by different persons. Now and then, among the earlier specimens of Berthelet's work, designs of a similar kind occur on the outside of the binding in gold, and inside the book printed in black. The occurrence of such a peculiarity would point strongly to the probability of the printer having also been the binder, or at all events that the control of both processes was in the hands of the same master.

Although no Mediæval English bindings of the richer sort are now left, several of the simpler kind bound in leather still remain. Most of these are ornamented with impressions from small cameo stamps impressed in blind,—that is to say, without gold. Most of such bindings are bound in dark brown leather, either goatskin, corresponding to our morocco, or sheepskin, corresponding to our roan. Each of these old leathers is sound and fine in colour, and always brown; colour dyes for leather, except red, being a later, and probably hurtful, innovation.

The boards of these bindings, like those of the decorated kind, are of wood, sometimes thick, sometimes thin. The thick boards were made heavy, because many of the manuscripts were written on vellum, which is very curly, and the weight of the covers was useful in counteracting this defect. The thin boards were very carefully chosen, and must have been well seasoned, as they are very rarely indeed warped at all. In many instances stamps of the monasteries at which they were made are impressed on these boards, and this is a sign of the careful manner in which even the smallest details concerning books was superintended. Berthelet's boards are always of cardboard or its equivalent, and although wooden boards are often found at a subsequent time to this, they may as a rule be considered to have gone out of universal use here about the end of the fifteenth century.

The reputed oldest specimen of all the English bookbindings is bound in red leather, possibly deerskin; it is known as "St. Cuthbert's Gospels," and was found, A. D. 1105, in the tomb of St. Cuthbert when it was opened. St. Cuthbert died A. D. 687, and the book is supposed to have been buried with him. It contains the Gospel of St. John, written on vellum, and is now treasured at Stonyhurst College. The volume is in such a remarkable state of preservation, both outside and inside, that a certain amount of discredit attaches to the legend of its great antiquity. It is bound in thin boards of limewood, covered with red leather, curiously worked and coloured. The upper cover bears a decorative rectangular panel, the central portion of which, nearly square, has a symmetrical foliated curve of double-S form, *repoussé*, and *showing* slight traces of colour; above and below this are two long panels in which are drawn free-hand scrolls of Anglo-Saxon character, deeply lined. These scrolls are painted blue and yellow. The under side is simply ornamented with fillets. The design of this binding is unquestionably very old, and may fittingly be referred to about the date of St. Cuthbert's death. Mr. E. Gordon Duff, however, inclines to the view that it is not actually the original binding, but is a copy of about the twelfth or thirteenth century. Even if it were made at the latest date attributed to it, it is still the earliest existing English book bound in red leather, as well as the only one decorated in the true style of Anglo-Saxon art.

Another early English book of great interest is a Latin Psalter of the eleventh century, in its original binding of thick oaken boards covered with brown leather. On each side is a sunk panel, and in one of these is a copper gilt figure of our Lord in the attitude of the crucifixion. The corners and clasp are of thin brass stamped with patterns, and are most likely of later date than the rest of the binding. A very interesting point about this book is, that it was used as the official coronation oath-book by all the English sovereigns from Henry I. to Henry VII.; it formerly belonged to the Exchequer, and was subsequently the property of the Marquis of Buckingham, who kept it in his beautiful library at Stowe; it is now in the British Museum.

With the exception of these two instances, all the English books bound in leather before the time of Thomas Berthelet are ornamented, if at all, with blind-stamped work only. In the cutting of stamps for this form of decoration, as well as in the designing of them, English artists in the twelfth century particularly are considered to have been superexcellent. The subject has been most ably and lucidly considered by Mr. James Weale, lately Art Librarian at the South Kensington Museum. He finds that such work was produced especially at Durham, Winchester, Oxford, and London, from the twelfth to the fifteenth centuries, after which there was such a marked irruption of foreign binders and foreign stamps that the English work became obscured, and on its recovery was of an entirely different character. But it is now generally conceded that these early English blind-tooled leather bindings are indeed the finest of the kind made anywhere.

The Winchester Domesday Book of the twelfth century, now belonging to the Society of Antiquaries of London, is a charming and typical specimen of this work; it is bound in dark brown goatskin, and ornamented with impressions in blind from beautifully cut small cameo stamps. The main scheme of the decoration is two large circles, one above the other, enclosed within a rectangular panel. The circles as well as the lines of the panel are curiously made up of successive impressions of small stamps. Those used in the circles are cut in such a manner that they can be used either separately or in combination. Used together, of course, certain stamps will only combine properly to form a circle of a particular

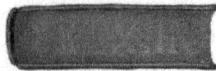

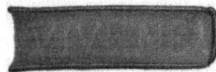

PLATE IV.

LEGEND WRITTEN ON THE EDGES OF A VOLUME OF
SIXTEENTH-CENTURY TRACTS. BOUND IN RED SATIN
FOR HENRY VIII.

circumference, as they are designed in short segments of circles, drop shaped, or in lozenge shapes, smaller at the base than at the top. It must be noted that the use of stamps cut in such a manner as to combine easily in circular forms is a characteristic of early English work. This circle, differently produced, however, will presently be seen again in Berthelet's designs, and it reappeared also in the seventeenth century on much of the remarkable work done on leather as well as on velvet, at the very interesting establishment founded at Little Gidding in Huntingdonshire by Nicholas Ferrar. Parts of circles are sometimes, but not often, found on the bindings made for Jean Grolier during the first half of the sixteenth century, but it is very seldom that the circle itself occurs as an integral part of the design on bookbindings. The circle as originally used in the artistic ornamentation of sculptures, goldsmiths' work, and the arts generally was probably a sun-sign. I fear bookbinding is not old enough to come under this ancient art influence very strongly; but it is just possible that the artists who designed the ornamentation of the leather covers of several of the splendid bindings made in England in Mediæval times, based largely upon the circle, and who cut their stamps so as easily to produce circles, may have been unconsciously following out the lines of thought inherited by them from artistic ancestors imbued with the ancient traditions. Crosses as well as circles are found sometimes on early leather bindings, but not in English work, and with these two exceptions I do not think any of the ancient symbols are represented in this particular line of art.

On the introduction of printing into England in the fifteenth century, the rich Mediæval bindings very rapidly became things of the past. The gap between them and the simple blind-stamped leather which rapidly superseded them was, however, filled to some extent by the production of very ornamental bindings in velvet and satin. These covers are mounted with bosses and clasps of precious metals and enamels, or embroidered in gold and ornamented with pearls. Several references and notes concerning such bindings occur in contemporary official documents, but no actual specimens now exist earlier than the time of Henry VII., but that king has left us several splendid examples.

Until Henry VIII. had his own royal binders, it is likely that all the early printers bound only their own work; but naturally a printer and binder holding an appointment as royal binder would be sometimes expected to bind other miscellaneous books, and instances of this are not only found in Berthelet's account, given below, but amongst the books bound by him there are some which were printed abroad and others which are collections of tracts, etc., all of which were bound for King Henry VIII. or his immediate successors.

The royal heraldry at the time Berthelet made his bindings was simple and dignified; first and fourth were the three fleurs-de-lys of France; second and third, the three lions of England. From William the Conqueror until Henry II., the royal coat of England probably consisted of two lions passant guardant in pale. Henry II., however, on his marriage with Eleanor, daughter of William V., Duke of Aquitaine and Guienne, incorporated the coat of that potentate, a single leopard, with his own, but as he probably considered the conjunction of this animal with those already on his coat might not be conducive to peace, he turned the leopard into a similar lion and added it to the others, and from that time the coat of arms of England has been "gules, three lions passant guardant in pale, or." The coat of France, "azure, semé de fleurs-de-lys, or," was adopted by Edward III., in the fourteenth year of his reign, together with the title of King of France, asserting his right to the coat and the title by virtue of his mother, Isabel, daughter of Philip IV. At first Edward placed the French coat in the second and third places of his shield, but presently gave it the places of honour, first and fourth, in consequence of a remonstrance from the French king. Edward's grandson, Richard II., married, as his second wife, Isabel, daughter of Charles VI. of France, who changed his coat, "semé de fleurs-de-lys," to one having only three fleurs-de-lys. Richard altered the French coat on his shield in accordance with this change, and this became the royal coat of arms of England until the accession of James I. With regard to the supporters which are found on some of Berthelet's bindings, they are only the dragon and the greyhound. The dragon is the red dragon of the last of the British kings, Cadwallader, from whom Henry VII. claimed descent, and in remembrance of whom he bore it as a supporter, as did all our Tudor sovereigns. This, however, is only one explanation, as it appears that a very similar badge was previously borne by Henry III., Edward I., and Edward III. The greyhound was also one of Henry VII.'s supporters, and is found on several of his bindings; it was used by Henry VIII. until about 1528, when he substituted a lion and changed the sides. This greyhound was borne by Henry VII. by a double right, partly by reason of his own descent from the Earls of Somerset, whose badge it was, and also by right of his wife through the Nevilles.

The badges found on Berthelet's bindings are the portcullis, used by all the Tudors in remembrance of the castle of the Beauforts in Anjou, where Henry VII.'s maternal grandfather was born; the double rose, red and white, used first by the Lancastrian Henry VII. on his marriage with Elizabeth of York, as a symbol of the union of the two rival houses; the fleur-de-lys, doubtless taken as one of the bearings from the French coat of arms; and the daisy, borne in remembrance of Margaret Beaufort, mother of Henry VII. All these are found on bindings made by Berthelet, sometimes singly and sometimes in combination on one binding.

Henry VII. was the first English king who attempted to form a library of his own, and besides manuscripts, he possessed a very fine collection of splendid volumes printed by Antoine Verard at Paris. These books are now part of the old Royal Library in the British Museum, and since they have been there they have all been rebound in velvet, which may probably be taken as some sign that they were originally bound in that material; and this is likely enough, as all the bindings still existing that belonged to this king are bound in it. Some of these beautiful bindings are now in the library at Westminster Abbey, but the finest example of any of them is in the British Museum.

During the reign of Henry VIII. some large heraldic panel stamps bearing the royal coat of arms were made here, probably by Dutch workmen, as they have characteristics of foreign workmanship. These stamps are often considered royal, but it is doubtful whether they ever were so. Two of them bear the royal coat of arms as used by Henry VII. and Henry VIII. One shows the royal coat, crowned, with supporters, stars, and a few flowers, and at the top the sun in glory and a half-moon with a face in profile, the arms of the City of London, and the cross of St. George; the other, a handsomer design, has likewise the royal coat of arms, crowned, with supporters, but at the top there are two angels carrying scrolls, and having between them a large double rose, while below are two portcullises, depending from the lower edge of the shield by chains. Two other panel stamps belonging to this series show the coats of arms of Queen Katharine of Aragon and Queen Anne Boleyn, and these have large shields, crowned, and supported by angels, with a ground on which are several flower sprays.

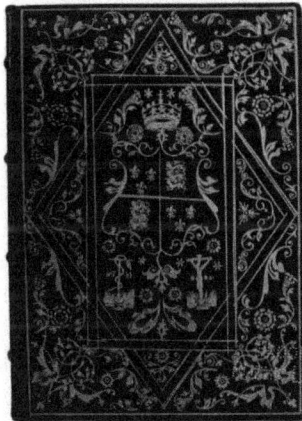

PLATE V.

CALF BINDING OF "GALTERI DELOENI LIBELLUS DE TRIBUS HIERARCHIIS." A MS. DEDICATED TO HENRY VIII., AND BOUND FOR HIM.

These stamps are always accompanied by another, which shows peculiar characteristics tending to prove that none of them are royal. This stamp always bears upon it some initial or device that belonged to a printer of the time. It consists of a large double rose supported by two angels, each bearing a scroll, on which, read together, is the legend, "*Hec rosa virtutis de celo missa sereno eternū florens regia sceptra feret.*" In the two upper corners are a sun in glory and a half-moon with face in profile, the shield of the City of London, the cross of St. George, and several stars. Below are a few scattered flower sprays and the initials or device of a printer. The commonest initials occurring on these panels are probably H. J., most likely Henry Jacobi; J. R., very likely John Reynes; G. G., possibly Garret Godfrey; R. L., perhaps Richard Lant; and many others of less note.

Judging from the use of the greyhound as one of the royal supporters, none of these stamps were cut after 1528, and Mr. Weale considers they may have been first used as early as 1485. I described and figured all of them in "The Queen" of June 20, 1891.

Although books bearing these designs are now generally considered non-royal, they are nevertheless frequently put forward as having belonged to Henry VII. and his successors, and in many places and catalogues they will be found so described. They are fine and well-cut stamps, and are impressed sometimes on sheep, but usually on fine calf leather; and no doubt if it were not for the existence upon them of trade-marks, private monograms, and city emblems, there would be much in favour of such a supposition. It may be that they were allowed to be used by members of the Stationers Company, at that time of much importance.

Immediately after the general discontinuance of large panel stamps with royal heraldic designs, Thomas Berthelet became royal printer and binder to Henry VIII., and the earliest of his large stamps bears some resemblance to the stamp just described as having two portcullises dependent from the lower part of the shield. It is possible that Berthelet took his design from this stamp. But whatever Berthelet's early bindings may have been like, the distinguishing characteristic of his work is the gold-tooling, properly so called, which he was, so far as is yet known, the first Englishman to use. A large portion of the printing he did was in the form of proclamations, single sheets, and other official matters, which were never bound; but as time went on, and the king, with his Tudor love of magnificence, perhaps to some extent regretting his own destruction of the beautiful and valuable Mediæval bindings, feeling that something more ornamental than the sombre panel stamps was wanted, Berthelet, being already royal printer, was no doubt further commissioned to make decorative royal bindings. This he did on both velvet and satin, materials already royal favourites, as well as using his new art of leather gilding in as decorative a manner as possible.

CHAPTER II.

DOCUMENTARY EVIDENCE CONCERNING BERTHELET AND HIS WORK.

It is evident that in the early part of the reign of Henry VIII. there was a large importation of foreign-bound books, much to the detriment of native workmen. So great was the abuse caused by this importation, that it was found advisable to issue various official papers on the subject.

The earliest English document concerning printed books is a statute made in the first year of King Richard III., by virtue of which foreigners were allowed to bring over their books and sell them without let or hindrance. The result of this permission was, however, not quite what was intended, as very shortly numbers of Englishmen became expert in the craft of printing "in all poyntes," as well as skilled in the "mysterye of byndynge"; and these found themselves so outnumbered by aliens and hampered by the foreign competition, that in 1533 an act was passed for their relief, the most important clause in which was one imposing a forfeit of six shillings and eight pence on every printed book brought from abroad ready bound in boards, leather, or parchment.

The act is as follows:—

"Anno XXV., Henrici VIII. (1533). Actis made in the session of this present Parliament, cap. XV. London, printed by Thomas Berthelet.

"Where as by the prouision of a statute made in the fyrste yere of the reygne of Kynge Rycharde the thyrde, it was prouided in the same acte, that all straungers repayrynge in to this realme, myghte laufully bringe in to the sayd realme printed and written bokes to selle at theyr libertie and pleasure. By force of whiche prouision there hath comen in to this realme sithen the makynge of the same, a maruelous nombre of printed bookes and daylye dothe. And the cause of the makynge of the same prouysion semethe to be, for that there were but fewe bokes and fewe printers with in this realme atte that tyme, whyche coulde welle exercise and occupie the sayd science and crafte of pryntynge: Never the lesse, sythen the makynge of the sayde prouisyon, manye of this realme, beynge the kynges naturalle subjectes, haue gyuen them soo delygentelye to lerne and exercyse the sayd crafte of printynge, that at this daye there be within this realme a greate nombre counnynge and experte in the sayd science or crafte of pryntynge, as able to exercyse the sayde crafte in all poyntes, as anye straunger in anye other realme or contray. And further more where there be a greate numbre of the kynges subiectes within this realme, whiche lyue by the crafte and mysterye of byndynge of books, and that there be a greate multitude welle experte in the same: yet all this not withstandynge there are dyuers persons, that bringe from beyonde the se greate plentie of printed bookes, not onelye in the latyne tonge, but also in our maternall englishe tonge some bounde in bordes, some in lether, and some in parchment, and them selle by retayle, wherby many of the kynges subiectes, beinge bynders of bokes, and hauing none other facultie wherewith to gette theyr lyuinge, be destitute of worke, and lyke to be vndone: except some reformation herin be had. Be it therefore enacted by the kynge oure soverayne lorde, the lordes spiritual and temporal, and the commons in this present parlyament assembled, and by auctoritie of the same, that the sayde Prouiso, made the fyrst yere of the sayd King Richarde the thirde from the feaste of the

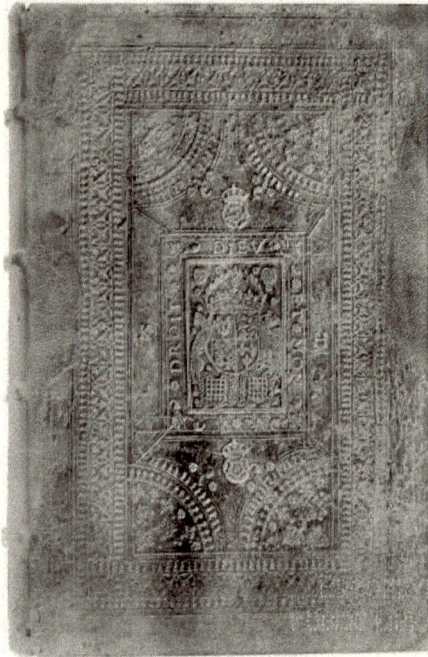

PLATE VI.

CALF BINDING OF A COPY OF THE WORKS OF ST. CHRYSOSTOM, PRINTED AT BASLE IN 1530. MADE FOR HENRY VIII.

natiuitie of our lorde god next commynge shalbe voyde and of none effecte. And further be it enacted by the auctorite afore sayde, that no person or persons, resiant or inhabitant within this realme after the sayd feast of Christmas next comyng shal bie to sel ageyne any printed bokes brought from any parties out of the kynges obeysance, redye bouden in bordes, lether, or parchement, uppon peyne to lose and forfayte for everye boke bounde oute of the sayde kynges obeysance, and brought into this realme, and bought by any person or persons within the same to sell agayne, contrarie to this act, syxe shyllynge eyghte pence.

"And be it further enacted by the auctorite afore-sayde, that no persone or persones inhabytant or resiante within this realme, after the saide feast of Christmas, shall bye within this realmes, of any stranger, borne oute of the kynges obedience other then of denizens, any manner of printed bokes, brought from any the parties beyond the see, except onely by engrose and not by retayle: upon peine of forfaiture of VI^s VIII^d for every boke so bought by retayle, contrarie to the fourme and effect of this estatute, the said forfaytures, to be always leuied of the byers of any suche bookes, contrarie to this act; etc. Provided alwaye, etc."

This act, stringent though it seems, was not of much effect, as presently appears by a study of the transcripts of the Stationers Company, most usefully reprinted by Mr. Edward Arber, amongst which will be found several rules and ordinations concerning the foreign bookbinders. These men, undoubtedly skilful in their trade, ultimately settled here in considerable numbers, and not only became naturalized Englishmen, but in all probability eventually benefited our styles and methods by the introduction of new ideas and a high standard of technical workmanship. A second great irruption of foreign workmen, binders among them, took place in England in 1685, on the revocation of the Edict of Nantes. On this occasion, also, it is probable that our native styles and methods ultimately benefited considerably by the importation of new blood.

Nothing is known about Thomas Berthelet until he became connected with the state printing under Henry VIII. He succeeded Richard Pynson as royal printer and binder in 1530, and received his appointment to this position by means of a royal patent. This patent is the earliest of the kind known, for although Pynson called himself "Printer unto the King's noble grace," his official authority for doing so is not forthcoming.

Berthelet's is, however, extant, and reads as follows:—

"Rex omnibus ad quos praesentes, ac, salutem. Sciatis quod nos de gratia nostra speciali, ac ex certa scientia, & mero motu nostris dedimus & concessimus, ac per praesentes damus et consedimus dilecto servienti nostro Thomae Barthelet impressori nostro quandam annuitatem, sive quendam annualem redditum quatuor librarum sterlingorum, habendum & annuatim percipiendum proedictam annuitatem sive annualem redditum quatuor librarum eidem Thomae Barthelet, à festo Paschae, anno regni nostro vicesimo primo, durante vita sua de thesauri nostro ad receptam scaccarii nostri per manus thesaurarum & camerarii nostrorum ibidem pro tempore existendo ad festa sancti Michaelis archangeli & Paschae per equales portiones &c., quod expressamentio &c. In cujus, &c. testimonium rei apud Westmonasteriensem, vicesimo secundo die Februarii, anno regni Henrici VIII., vicesimo primo. Per breve privato sigillo."

It will be seen that by virtue of this document Berthelet enjoyed a life income of four pounds sterling annually, the same sum that had been given to Richard Pynson in September, 1515. There is also a note to this effect among the Patent Rolls. (21 Hen. VIII., Pt. II. m. 17, dated York Place 13th Feby 21 Hen. VIII.)

Not only was he thus marked for the king's favour, but he also enjoyed what in those days was considered a high honour; he was granted a coat of arms by Clarenceulx, king of arms, on September 1, 1549. This grant exists in the College of Arms in London, and the arms are thus described:—

"The armes and creste of Thomas Berthelet of London, esquyer, gentillman; he bereth asure on a cheveron flore contre flore argent, betwene three doves of the same, thre trefiles vert. per chrest. upon his helm, out of a crounall silver two serpents endorsed asure ventred gold open mouthed, langued and eyed geules, there tailes comyng up in saulre under thire throtes, the endes of the tailes entering into their eres, langued and armed geules manteled geules, doubled silver, as more plainly apperith depicted in this margent; graunted and given by me Thomas Hawley alias Clarenceulx, Kyng of armes, the first day of September in the thirde yere of the reygne of our soverange lorde Kynge Edward the VI etc."

Pynson used heraldic emblems with the helmet of an esquire on some of his bindings; but he appears to have assumed the dignity without official warrant.

Berthelet's continued presence in England was also considered of sufficient importance to justify a special exemption in his favour from serving the king abroad in his wars in France. (Patent Roll. 36 Hen. VIII., Pt. II.)

In the state papers preserved in the Record Office in London are several notices referring to the official printing work done by Thomas Berthelet. These testify to the importance and confidential nature of the work intrusted to him, and show how he was sometimes, on particularly urgent or secret occasions, ordered to set up the type himself, and also was obliged to take an oath of secrecy. Misprints were evidently a thorn in his side, more than one entry referring to such difficulties, of which doubtless numbers escaped official notice. From these entries I have chosen a few for quotation.

Treasurer of the Chamber's Accounts.

Oct 22nd 1530. To Thos Bartlet (Berthelet) for printing 1600 papers and books of proclamation for ordering and punishing sundry beggars and vacabundes, and dampnyng of books containing certain errors, at 1d per leaf. £8 6s 8d.

(Trevelyan Papers. Record Office. Letters and Papers Hen. 8th Vol. 5. p. 322.)

Richard Croke to Cromwell 17th Septr. 1532.

After I left, Bartelot, the printer, told me that Goodrycke requested him to advertise the King of certain errors in "The Glasse off Truthe," which Bartelot refused, saying he had moved the King in such matters beforetime, and his Grace was not content with it. Though this was told Croke secretly, thinks it his duty to make it known to Cromwell, and that he should get out by policy from Goodricke what errors he notes. Thinks that Bartelot will speak of it to others.

(Letters and Papers Hen. 8th Vol. 5. No. 1320. p. 572.)

Cromwell to Sir Thomas Audeley, Lord Chancellor. 11th Novr. 1534.

It is necessary to have some copies of the proclamation printed to night, that they may be sent to sundry parts with the books of answer. Desires him to send a true copy by the bearer. Will then send for Bartelet the printer, swear him and cause him to have them printed to-night. The Rolls, 11 Nov.

Asks him to have the proclamations written and sealed, and bring them to-morrow at 10 o'clock. The duke of Norfolk and he will tarry dinner till he comes.

Below is Audeley's answer.

Will have 20 proclamations written as Cromwell wishes. Has commanded Crooke to deliver one true original to Bartelott with orders to set the print himself to-night, and make speed. Will be with Cromwell to-morrow at the hour appointed.

(Letters and Papers Hen. 8th Vol. 7. p. 535. No. 1415.)

The most important as well as the most interesting document concerning Berthelet is a long bill of his, giving details of books supplied by him to King Henry VIII., between the dates 1541-1543. This bill is written on twelve leaves of paper, and with it a warrant on vellum, signed by the king, ordering the payment to be made. Berthelet's autograph receipt is also appended. This document was purchased by the British Museum in 1870, and although it does not seem that any of the items mentioned in it can positively be identified, there are many instances in which it is likely enough that in the same museum are some of the actual books referred to. (Add. MS. 28. 196.)

Several of the entries in this bill are of great interest. We find that many of the bindings were bound back to back; none now remain that were made at so early a date, but several instances of this curious method of binding that were made during the seventeenth century, bound both in leather and in satin, still exist.

White leather "gorgiously gilted on the leather" is mentioned more than once, and velvet, purple, and black were occasionally used, but the style of the decoration of it is left entirely to the imagination.

Again, "Crymosyn satin" only is mentioned, without any word of embroidery or other ornamentation, while leather, probably brown calf, is here and there described as being "gorgiously gilte," and also "bounde after the Italian" or "Venecian fascion."

The prices in this bill should be multiplied by about twelve to bring them into line with our present currency.

The bill is worded as follows:—

We wolle and commaunde you that of suche our Treausour as in your handes remayneth ye doe ymedyatly upon the sighte herof pay or doe to be paide unto our trustie servaunte Thomas Berthelett our prynter the somme of one hundred seventene pounds sixepence and one halfepeny sterlyng. The whiche is due and owyng by us unto hym for certeyne parcelles delyvered by the seid Thomas unto us and other at our commandement as in this booke, whereunto this our present warraunte is annexed particularly dothe appere. And these our lettres signed with our hande shalbe unto you a suffycient warraunte and discharge for the same. Yoven under our Signemanuell, at our Manour of Wodstooke, the xxiiij^{tl} of September, the xxxv yere of our reigne.

To our right trustie and righte welbeloved Sr. Edward Northe, Knyghte, treausourer of thaugmentaciouns of the Revenues of our Crowne.

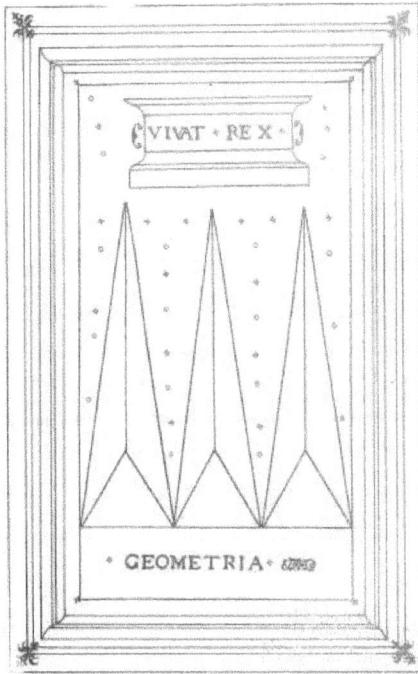

VIVAT · RE X

· GEOMETRIA ·

PLATE VII.

WHITE LEATHER BINDING OF A MS. ENTITLED "LA
SCIENCE DE GEOMETRIE."

*Receyved of sir Edward North, Knight, treasourer of the Augmentations, the sayd summe
of one hundred seventene poundes vj. d. ob. according to the tenour of this warrant, the 29
day September, a° regni regis Henrici viij, xxxv.*

Anno Domini 1541, et anno regni serenissimi et invictissimi Regis Henrici
Octavi, Dei gratia Anglie Francie et Hibernie Regis, fidei Defensoris, et in
terra Ecclesie Anglicane et Hibernice Supremi Capitis, tricesimo tercio.

In primis, delyvered to my Lorde Chaumcellour, the ixth day of December,
xx^{ti} Proclamacons, made for the enlargyng of Hatfeld Chace, printed in fyne
velyme, at vj^{d} the pece. Summa, 10s.

Item delyvered to the Kinges hyghnes, the xxx day of December, a Newe
Testament in englisshe and latyn, of the largest volume, price 3s.

Item delyvered to the Kinges hyghnes, the vj day of January, a Psalter in englisshe and latyne, covered with crimoysyn satyne, 2s.

Item delyvered the same tyme, a Psalter, the Proverbes of Salomon, and other smalle bookes bounde together, price 16d.

Item delyvered to the Kinges hygnes, for a little Psalter, takyng out of one booke and settyng in an other in the same place, and for gorgious byndyng of the same booke, xijd and to the Goldesmythe, for taking of the claspes and corner, and for settyng on the same ageyne xvjd Summa 2s. 4d.

Item delyvered unto the Kinges hyghnes, the xv day of January, a New Testament in latyne, and a Psalter englisshe and latyne, bounde backe to backe, in white leather, gorgiously gilted on the leather; the bookes came to ijS. the byndyng and arabaske drawyng in golde on the transfile, iiijs Summa 6s.

Item delyvered to the Kinges hyghnes, the xviij day of January, a booke called *Enarraciones Evangeliorum Dominicalium*, bounde in crymosyn satyne; the price 3s. 4d.

Item delyvered to the Kinges hig(h)nes, the xxiij day of January, a booke of the Psalter in englisshe and latyne, the price viijd; and a booke entiteled *Enarraciones Evangeliorum Dominicalium*, the price xijd; and for the gorgious byndyng of them, backe to backe, iijs iiijd Summa 5s.

Item delyvered to Maister Hynwisshe, to the Kinges use, a paper booke of vj queres royall, gorgiously bounde in leather 7s. 6d.

Item delyvered to my Lorde Chauncellour, the xxv day of January vjc. Proclamacions concernyng the Kinges stile; eche of them conteynyng one leafe of bastarde paper, at jd the pece. Summa 50s

Item delyvered to my Lorde Chauncellour, the iiij day of February, vjc. Proclamacions concernyng eatyng of whyte meates; eche of them conteyning one hole leafe of Jene paper, at ob. the pece, 25s

Item delyvered the xxvth day of February, to the Kinges hyghnes, *Ambrosius super epistolas sancti Pauli xxd*

Item one Psalter in englisshe, in viijo xxd.

Item ij litle Psalters, xvjd Summa 4s. 8d.

Item delyvered to the Kinges hyghnes, the laste day of February, xij bookes intitled *Summaria* (in) *Evangelia et Epistolas ut leguntur*, ij bounde in paper bordes at viijd the pece, and x in forrelles, at vjd the pece, 6s. 4d.

Item delyvered to the Kinges hyghnes, the iij day of Marche, one *Summaria in Evangelia et Epistolas*, gorgiously bounde, and gilte on the leather, price 2s.

Item delyvered the same day, ij bookes, intitled *Conciliaciones locorum Althemeri*, price 4s.

Item delyvered to the Kinges hyghnes, the same day, one *Opus Zmaragdi*, price 4s. 8d.

Item delyvered to the Kinges hyghnes, the vth day of Marche, one *Novum Testamentum*, bounde with a *Summaria*, price 2s.

Item delyvered to the Kinges hyghnes, the ix day of Marche, one *Novum Testamentum*, in latyne, bounde with a *Summaria super Epistolas et Evangelia*, 2s.

Item delyvered to the Kinges hyghnes, the xij^t day of Marche, one *Authoritas allegabiles sacre scripture*, with one *Summaria in Evangelia et Epistolas*, gorgiously bounde in whyte, and gilte on the lether, iiij Item, *Sedulius in Paulum* at iijs. Item, *Petrus Lumberdus in Epistolas sancti Pauli*, at iij^s iiij^d. Item, *Homelie ven. Bede in Epistolas Dominicalis*, at xvj^d. Item, *Questiones Hugonis super Epistolas sancti Pauli*, ij$ₛ$ Summa 13s. 8d.

Item delyvered to the Kinges Maiestie, the xv day of Marche, *Thomas de Aquino, in Evangelia Dominicalia, et Homelie Bede, una ligati cum alijs*; price 2s 8d.

Item, *Psalterium* in latyne, and a Psalter in englisshe, *una legati*; price 2s. 8d.

Item, *Arnobius super psalmos*, 2s.

Item, *Haymo super psalmos*, 2s.

Item, *Jo, de Turre-cremata super Evangelia*, 2s 8d.

Item, *Omelia Haymonis super Evangelia*, 16d.

Item delyvered to the Kinges hyghnes, the xvj day of Marche, one *Arnobius super Psalterium*, bounde with other bookes, 2s.

Item, delyvered to the Kinges hyghnes, the xviij day of Marche, one *Arnobius super Psalterium*, and one Psalter in englisshe, price 2s. 8d.

Item delyvered to the Kinges hyghnes, the xix day of Marche, *Homilie Bede hyemales*, bounde with his *Homilijs on the Pistles*, price 2s. 8d.

Item, *Homilie Bede aestivales*, bound alone, price 20d.

Item delyvered to the Kinges hyghnes, the xxiij day of Marche, *Homelie Bede pars estivalis*, bounde with his Homilies on the Epistoles, price 2s. 8d.

Item the same day, delyvered to his grace, *Enarraciones sancti Thome de Aquino super Evangelia*, bounde with *Homilijs Bede super Epistolas*, the price 2s. 8d.

Anno Domini 1542.

Item delyvered to the Kinges hyghnes, the xxv^{ti} day of Marche, one Psalter in latyne of Colines printe, and one in englisshe, bounde together; the price ij^s viii^d. Item, *Arnobius super Psalterium*, and a Psalter in englisshe, bound together, price ij^s viij^d. Item, *San(c)tus Thomas de Aquino super Mathuem*, the price ij^s. Summa 6^s 8^d

Item delyvered to the Kinges hyghnes, the xxvij day of Marche, one *Cathena aurea divi Thome de Aquino in Evangelia Dominicalia*, price ij iiij^d.

Item the same day delyvered to his hyghnes, one *Postilla Guilielmi Par(is)iensis*, price ijş Summa 5s. 4d.

Item delyvered to the Kinges hyghnes, the xxviij dau of Marche, one *Enarraciones sancti Thome de Aquino in Evangelia Dominicalia, with Homilijs ven. Bede in Epistolas ut per totum annum leguntur in templis*, price ij^s viij^d. Item, *Psalterium* in latine, with *Arnobius super Psalmos*; the price ij^s viij^d. Item, *Faber super Epistolas Catholicas* the price xx^d. Item, *Dydimus Alexandrianus*, with Beda upon the *Epistolas Catholicas*, price ij^s. Item, one *Catanus super Evangelia*, price iij^s iiij^d Summa 12s.

Item delyered to the Kinges hyghnes, the xxx day of Marche, one *Cathena Aurea divi Thome Super Evangelia in duobos*, price 5s.

Item delyvered the same day to his grace, one *Dionysius Carth.*; and a *Faber Stampe super Epistolas Catholicas*, price 3s.

Item delyvered the same day, one *Dydimus Alexandrinus*, and *Beda super Epistolas Catholicas*, price 2s.

Item delyvered to the Kinges hyghnes, the ij day of Aprill, one *Thomas de Aquino in Evangelia Dominicalia*, and *Beda super Epistolas*, bounde together, price 2s 8d.

Item delyvered to the Kinges hyghnes, the same day, one *Homilie Johannis Chrysostomi in Matheum*, the price 2s.

Item, one *Homilie Jo. Chrysostomi in Johannem Marcum et Lucam*, price 2s. 4d.

Item delyvered to the Kinges hyghnes, the xj^t day of Aprill, *Dionysium Carthus. in Evang.* in viij, bound in ij, price 5s.

Item delyvered the same day, to my Lorde Chauncellour of England, iiij^c Proclamacions concernyng stealyng of haukes egges, and kepyng of soure haukes; eche conteynyng a leafe of basterde paper, at j^d the pece. Summa 35s.

Item delyvered to my Lorde Chauncellour the xvj day of Aprill, iiij^c Proclamacions concernyng stealing of haukes eggs, and kepyng of soure haukes; eche of them conteynyng a hole leaffe of Jene paper at ob. the pece. Summa 16s. 8d.

Item for iiij^c of the same, that were new made ageyne, at ab. the pece. Summa 16s. 8d.

Item delyvered to my Lorde Chauncellour of England, the xx day of Aprill, all these Actes foll),owyng, printed in Proclamacions; that is to wete, v^c of the Acte concernyng counterfeit lettres or privie tokens, to receyve money or goodes in other mens handes; eche of them conteynyng a leaffe of Jene paper, at ob. the pece, 20s. 10d.

Item delyvered v^c of the Acts concernyng bying of fisshe upon the see; eche of them conteyning one hole leaffe of basterde paper, at j^d the pece. Summa 41s. 8d.

Item delyvered ij^c of the Acte concernyng foldyng of clothes in North Walles, eche of them conteynyng halfe a leaffe of basterde paper, at ob. the pece. Summa 8s. 4d.

Item v^c of the Acte concernyng pewterers; eche of them conteynyng one hole leaffe of basterde paper, at j^d ob. the pece. Summa 3l. 2s. 6d.

Item C of the Acte concernyng kepyng of greate horsses; eche of them conteynyng ij hoole leafes of basterde paper, at ij^d the pece. Summa 4l. 3s. 4d.

Item V^c of the Acte concernyng crossboues and hande gonnes; eche of them conteynyng iij holle leaves dim. of basterde paper at iiij^d ob. the pece. Summa 7l. 5s. 10d.

Item V^c of the Acte concernyng the conveyaunce of brasse, latene, and bell metall over the see; eche of them conteynyng one holle leafe of basterde paper, at j^d the pece. Summa 41s. 8d.

Item v^c of the Acte ageynst conjuracions, witchecraftes sorcery, and inchauntementes eche of them conteynyng one holle leafe of Jene paper, at ob. the pece. Summa 20s. 10d.

Item v^c of the Acte for the mayntenaunce of artillarie, debarryng unlaufull games; eche of them conteynyng iiij holle leaves of basterde paper, at lllj^d the pece. Summa 8l. 6s. 8d.

Item v^c of the Acte concernyng the execucion of certeyne Statutes; eche of them conteynyng iij hoole leaves dim. of bastarde paper, at iiij^d ob. the pece. Summa 7l. 5s. 10d.

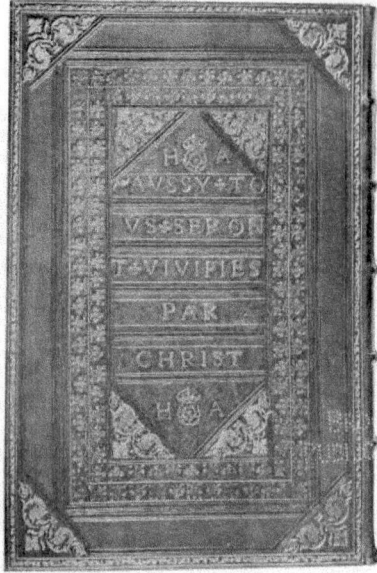

PLATE VIII.

UPPER COVER OF THE CALF BINDING OF VOL. I. OF A
BIBLE PRINTED AT ANTWERP IN 1534. MADE FOR HENRY
VIII. AND QUEEN ANNE BOLEYN.

Item v^c of the Acte for bouchers to selle at their libertie, by weyghte or otherwise; eche of them conteynyng one holle leafe of basterde paper, at 1^d the pece. 41s. 8d.

Item v^c of the Acte for murdre and malicius bloudshed within the Courte; eche of them conteynyng iiij hole leaves dim. of Basterde paper at iij^d ob. the pece. Summa 7l. 5s. 10d.

Item xij of the Acte concernyng certeyne Lordships, translated from the Countie of Denbigh to the Countie of Flynt; eche of them conteynyng one hoolle leaffe of basterde paper, at j^d the pece. Summa 12d.

Item v^c of the Acte concernyng false prophesies upon declaracion of armes, names, or badges; eche of them conteynyng a dim. leafe of basterde paper, at ob. the pece, 20s. 10d.

Item v^c of the Acte concernyng the translation of the saynctuarie from Manchestere to Westechester; eche of them conteynyng one hoolle leaffe dim. of basterde paper, at j^d ob. the pece. Summa 3l. 2s. 6d.

Item v^c of the Acte for worsted yarne in Northefolke; eche of them conteynyng a hoolle leaffe of basterde paper, at j^d the pece. Summa 41s. 8d.

Item v^c of the Acte for confirmacion and continuacion of certeyne Actes; eche of them conteynyng one hoolle leafe of basterde paper, at j^d the pece. Summa 41s. 8d.

Item v^c of the Acte for the true making of kerseyes; eche of them conteynyng one holle leafe dim, of basterde paper, at j^d ob. the pece. Stmma 3l. 2s. 6d.

Item v^c of the Acte expondyng a certeyn Statute concernyng the shippyng of clothes; eche of them conteynyng a dim leafe of basterde paper, at ob. the pece. Summa 20s. 10d.

Item for the byndyng of ij Primmers, written and covered with purple velvet, and written abowte with golde, at iij^s the pece. Summa 6s.

Item delyvered to the Kinges hyghnes, the vj day of Maye, xij of the Statutes made in the Parliament holden in the xxxiij^{ti} yere of his moste gracious reigne; at xvj^d the pece. Summa 16s.

Item delyvered to Mr James, Maister Denes servaunte for the Kinges hyghnes use, the xvjth day of Maye, a greate booke of paper imperiall, bound after the facion of Venice, price 15s.

Item delyvered to the seid Maister James, for the Kinges hyghnes use, another greate booke of paper imperiall, bounde after the Italian fascion, the price 14s.

Item delyvered the xiiij day of June, to Maister Daniell, servaunte to Maister Deny, to the Kinges hyghnes use, ij bookes of paper royall, bound after the Venecian fascion, the price, 18s.

Item delyvered to Maister Secretory, Maister Wrysley the v day of November, iij dosen bookes of the Declaracion of the Kinges hyghnes title to the soverayntie of Scotland, at iiij^d the pece. Summa 12s.

Item delyvered to Maister Jones, servaunte to Maister Deny, the xxx daye of December, v *Tullius de Officijs*, bounde in paper bourdes, at xvj^d the pece, and one gorgiously gilted for the Kinges hyghnes, price iij^s iiij^d Summa, 10s.

Item for byndyng of a paper booke for the Kinges hyghnes, and the gorgious giltyng thereof, delyvered the xiiij day of January to Mr Turner, 3s. 4d.

Item delyvered to Maister Hynnige, for the Kinges hyghnes use the vij day of Febr. a greate paper booke of royall paper, bounde after the Venecian fascion, price 8s.

Item delyvered the ix day of February, to my Lorde Chauncellour, vj^c of the Proclamacions for white meates, at ob. the pece, 25s.

Item delyvered the vj day of Marche, iij bookes of "The Institution of a xp'en man," made by the clergy, vnto the Kinges most honerable Counsayll at xx^d the pece, 5s.

Anno Domini 1543.

Item delyvered the vj day of Aprill, to Maister Henry Knyvett, for the Kinges hyghnes, a bridgement of the Statutes, gorgiously bounde, 5s.

Item delyvered to the Kinges moost honerable Counsaill, the viiij day of Aprill, iij litle bookes of the Statutes, price xij^d Item iij bookes of the vj Articles, price vj^d Item iij of the Proclamacions ageynst Anabaptistes, price vj^d Item iij Proclamacions of ceremones, price vj^d Item iij of the Injunccions, price vj^d Item iij of holy dayes, price iij^d Summa. 3s. 3d.

Item delyvered to my Lorde Chauncellour of England the iiij daye of Maye, ij^c Proclamacions concernyng the price of suger, conteynyng one hole leafe of basterde paper, at j^d the pece. Summa. 16s. 8d.

Item for the byndyng of a booke written on vellim, by Maister Turner, covered with blacke velvet, 16d.

Item delyvered to my Lorde Chauncellor, the xxxj day of Maye, v^c of the Acte for the advauncement of true religion and abolisshment of the contrarie, made out in Proclamacions; eche of them conteynyng iii leaves dim. of greate basterde paper, at iijd. ob. the pece. Summa, 7l. 5s. 10d.

Item delyvered v^c of the Acte for the explanacion of the statutes of willes, made out in Proclamacions; eche of them conteynyng iii leaves of great basterd paper, at iijd the pece. Summa, 6s. 5d.

Item delyvered v^c of the Acte agaynst suche parsones as doe make bankeruptes, made out in Proclamacions, eche of them conteynyng two greate leaves of basterde paper, at ijd. the pece. Summa, 4l. 3s. 4d.

Item delyvered v^c of the Acte for the preservacion of the ryver of Severne, made oute in Proclamacions; eche of them conteynyng two small leaves of paper, at jd, the pece; 41s. 8d.

Item delyvered v^c of the Acte concernyng collectours and receyvours, made out in Proclamacions; eche of them conteyning a leafe dim. of paper, at jd. the pece. Summa, 41s. 8d.

Item delyvered v^c of the Acte for the true making of coverlettes in Yorke, made oute in Proclamacions; eche of them conteyning ij smalle leaves of paper, at jd. the pece. Summa. 41s. 8d.

Item delyvered v^c of the Acte for the assise of cole and woode, made owt in Proclamacions; eche of them conteynyng a leafe of smalle paper, at ob. the pece. Summa, 20s. 10d.

Item delyvered v^c of the Acte, that persons, beyng noe common surgions, may mynistre outwarde medycines, made oute in Proclamacions; eche of them conteynyng a leafe of smalle paper, at ob. the pece. Summa, 20s. 10d.

Item delyvered v^c of the Acte to auctorise certeyne of the Kinges majesties counsaill to sett prices upon wines; made out in Proclamacions, eche of them conteynyng a leafe of paper, at ob. the pece. Summa, 20s. 10d.

Item delyvered v^c of the Acte for the true making of pynnes, made out in Proclamacions; eche of them conteynyng halfe a leafe of paper, at ob. the pece. Summa, 10s 5d ½d.

Item delyvered v^c of the Acte for the true making of frises and cottons in Wales, made oute in Proclamacions; eche of them conteynyng a leafe of paper, at ob. the pece. Summa, 21s. 8d.

Item delyvered fiftie of the Acte for pavying of certeyne lanes

PLATE IX.

SATIN BINDING OF A COLLECTION OF SIXTEENTH-CENTURY TRACTS. MADE FOR HENRY VIII.

and streets in London and Westm., made out in Proclamacions; eche of them conteynyng ij leaves of smalle paper, at jd. the pece, 4s. 2d.

Item delyvered fiftie of the Acte for knyghtes and burgeses to have places in the parliament, for the county-palantyne and citie of Chester, made out in Proclamacions; eche of them conteynyng a leaffe of smalle paper, at ob. the pece; 2s. 1d.

Item delyvered fourtie bookes of the Acte for certeyne ordenaunces in the Kinges majesties dominion and principalitie of Wales, at iiij^d the pece. Summa 13s. 4d.

Item delyvered to the Kinges highnes, the firste day of June, xxiiij bookes intitled "A necessary doctrine for any Christen man," at xvjd. the pece. Summa, 32s.

Item delyvered to the Kinges hyghnes, the third day of June xxiiij bookes intitled "A necessary doctrine for any Christen man," at xvj^d the pece. Summa, 32s.

Item delyvered to the Kinges hyghnes, the iiij day of June, xxiiij of the booke intitled "A necessary doctryne for any Christen man," at xvjd the pece. Summa, 32s.

Item delyvered to Maister Stokeley, the xij day of June, xij Proclamacions for the advancement of true religion, at iijd. ob. the pece; 3s. 6d.

Item xx of the Proclamacions of the Acte for explanacion of the statute of willes, at iijd the pece. Summa, 5s.

Item xj proclamacions of the Acte of bankerupte, at ijd. the pece. Summa, 3s. 4d.

Item xx Proclamacions of the Acte for Severne, at jd. the pece. Summa, 20d.

Item xx Proclamacions of the Acte of collectours and receyvours, at jd, the pece, 20d.

Item xx Proclamacions of the Acte for making of coverlettes in Yorke, at jd. the pece. Summa, 20d.

Item xx of the Proclamacions, that persones beyng noe comon surgions may ministre outewarde medicynes, at ob. the pece. Summa, 10d.

Item xx Proclamacions of the Acte for certeyne of the Kinges maiesties counsaill to sett prices of wynes; at ob. the pece. Summa, 10d.

Item xx Proclamacions of the Acte for true making of pynnes, at q^a the pece, 5d.

Item xx Proclamacions of the Acte for true making of frises and cottons in Wales; at ob. the pece. Summa, 10d.

Summa totalis, cxvijli vj. d. ob.

THOMAS AUDELEY,
Cancellarius.

The consideration of Thomas Berthelet as a printer is foreign to my present purpose; the subject is a large one, and requires special treatment and a long and careful study. There are more works left that were printed by Berthelet than there are of any other of our early English printers, and the greater number of the works he chose for reproduction are important and valuable,—147 books are known to have been printed by him. Many of Berthelet's types are very beautiful. Some of them are black letter; perhaps one of the finest founts is that used for the Confessio Amantis of John Gower. Plate II. shows a reproduction of the beautiful title-page of this book, of which I believe the border is one of Berthelet's own designing, or at all events made by the design of the stamps used on his bindings; the resemblance of many of the black curves printed in this book to those used in gold on the leather will be at once apparent. Whenever any student ventures upon a close examination of the printed work of Berthelet, he will be met with an important initial difficulty, which is, that Berthelet's nephew and successor, Thomas Powell, was misguided enough to leave out the word "late" on several of his imprints; that is to say, he printed many books absolutely as if they had been issued by Berthelet himself, using the same types and the same trade expressions altogether. In many instances it will be almost impossible to decide definitely whether a particular book was printed by the master himself or only by his man.

In the long list of works printed by Berthelet which is given by Ames, there are statutes dated as early as 1529; and besides official publications, there are numerous miscellaneous books of an important character. Among these are several written by Sir Thomas Elyot and Erasmus; Gower's Confessio Amantis; Lyttylton's Tenures; bibles, dictionaries, plays, and chronicles.

On the title-page of a copy of Marcus Aurelius's golden book is an ornamental border. This border consists of a design of boys in procession, one being carried on the shoulders of four others, and has at the top a medallion with two sphinxes; the same design, however, if not the same block, was used by other printers besides Berthelet. Berthelet's own device is a figure of Lucretia stabbing herself, with a landscape in the distance and an architectural framework.

The colophons in Berthelet's books are found both in Latin and in English, one of the most usual being:—

"Imprinted in Fletestrete in the house of Thomas Berthelet nere to the condite at the sygne of Lucrece."

Common forms are also:—

"Londoni in Aedibus Tho. Bertheleti," "Thome Bertheletus regius impressor excudebat," and "Impressus Londini in edibus regii impressoris."

And of rarer occurrence are the words:—

"In Aedibus Thome. Bertheleti typographi regii typis impress," and "Impressum in Flete-Strete prope aquagium sub intersignio Lucretiae Romanae."

There is a curious limit given as to price in a note at the end of a copy of the "Doctrine and Erudition for any Christian Man," printed in 1543, which says: "This boke bounde in paper boordes or claspes, not to be sold aboue XVI^d."

A few books were printed from 1556 to 1560 with Berthelet's colophons, after his death, on which the word "late" is prefixed to his name, but this does not appear always to have been done.

Thomas Berthelet enjoyed what in his time must have been a very lucrative post. Not only had he his regular fee, but he was also constantly employed in official work, for which he was separately paid, besides which he had private customers. There are several entries respecting the investment of his property to be found in the Patent Rolls of Henry VIII. Among these there are some which are of interest, as showing how carefully changes of property were noted in those days; e. g.:—

"On payment of a sum of 40 shillings licence was granted to Richard Moryson to alienate two houses in Friday Street to Thomas Berthelet." (Patent Roll. 34 Hen. VIII., Pt. II.)

Again: "Grant to Thomas Berthelet of messuages and lands in St. Andrews, Holborn, and St. Bride's Fleet Street for a sum of £189. 3. 11." (Patent Roll. 35 Hen. VIII., Pt. III.)

And yet another grant is found in the Patent Roll, 36 Henry VIII., Pt. XII., by which Thomas Berthelet received the following property in consideration of a payment of £212. 10. 0.:—

"A house in the parish of St. Bride, known as Salisbury Place formerly in the occupation of Richard Hyde, and before that belonging to the dissolved monastery of Godstowe in Oxfordshire.

"A house in the parish of St. Margaret Moyses in Friday Street in the city of London in the occupation of John Stanes.

"Another house in the same parish in the occupation of James Wilson, and various houses also in the same parish in the occupation of William Egleston.

"A house in Distaff Lane in the parish of St. Margaret Moyses in the occupation of John Greene.

"All the above houses in the parish of St. Margaret's having formerly belonged to the monastery of the Graces near the Tower of London.

"Two houses in the parish of St. Bride, Fleet Street, one in the occupation of John Hulson (scriptoris) and the other in the occupation of John Lyons goldsmith (aurifabri), both of which were previously part of the possessions of the Priory and Hospital of St. John of Jerusalem."

The will of Thomas Berthelet, Citizen and Stationer of London, is dated September 23, 1555. It directs that his property shall be chiefly divided between his wife Margery and his two sons, Edward and Anthony, to each of whom substantial property in land and houses is left, the elder one receiving the manor of Hilhampton in Hereford.

Thomas Powell, his nephew, and all his godchildren are remembered, also his wife's sister; and each apprentice receives the value of his own yearly royal fee, four pounds.

The will also—

Directs that his body shall be buried in the parish church of St. Bride's, Fleet Street, in the Lady Chapel, and gives to his Son and heir, Edward Barthelett, the manor of Hilhampton alias Ilhampton, in the Co. of Hereford, and land in Marden, messuages and tenements in Fleet Street, Bishopsgate Street, and Friday Street, amounting in all to one third of his estate.

To his Younger Son, Anthony Barthelett, he leaves premises in Distaff Lane, Friday Street, Bread Street, St. Sepulchre's parish, St. Andrews, Holborn, with reversion to elder brother, and Thomas Powell, his nephew.

To his Wife, Margaret (Margery), he gives property in the parish of St. Andrews, Holborn,

"and the house with the ways walks etc, which I reserve for my own use in Crokhorne Alley in the said parish of St. Andrews,"

—and a house in the parish of St. Sepulchre, with reversion to the two sons and the heirs of Margery, his wife.

His goods to be divided into three parts, one to go to his wife, the second to his two sons, with reversion to Christ's Hospital, "*lately erected.*" The third part reserved to pay funeral expenses and provide the following:—

- To Thomas Powell, "nephew," £40 in goods.

- "Prudence Skynner, goddaughter, 20 shillings.

- "Martha Salvoine, goddaughter, 20 shillings.

- "each of his other godchildren six and eightpence.

- "the church box at St. Bride, 20 shillings.

- "Christ's Hospital, ten pounds.

- "Alice Cowper, wife's sister, four pounds in money.

- "each of his apprentices, four pounds in money or money's worth.

- "son Edward, gold chain weighing 12 ozs.

- " " "Anthony, gold chain weighing 7 ozs.

- Residue of goods left to wife, Margery, sole executrix.

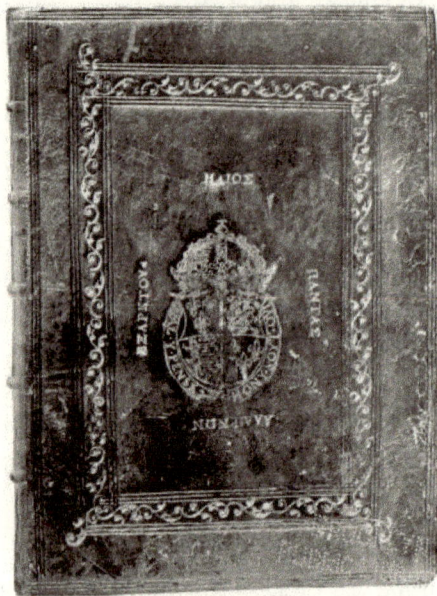

PLATE X.

CALF BINDING OF "JUL. CLAUD IGUINI ORATIO AD HEN. VIII." MADE FOR THE KING.

Trustees, John Abingtone, gentleman, clerk of the Queen's woodyard, and John Wekes, citizen and goldsmith, with a legacy of four pounds apiece.

Witnesses, Richard Heywood.

Edward Ridge.

John Hulson.

Probate granted 9th Novr 1555.

He probably died shortly after this will was executed, as there is the following entry in the Stationers' Hall Book A, of the date 1556: "Rec^d of Margery barthelett wydow XXVI Janu. iij^l vl^s viij^d which Tho. Berthelett hyr husbande receuyed of Mr. Chamberlayne to the use of our companye for Mr. andrewes Rewarde at his settynge over to the vyntenners.... Item recevyd at the presente tyme of the sayde margery for a rewarde to the cōpanye for comynge to the sayde thomas bartheletts his buryal xiii iiij."

Mrs. Margery eventually married Richard Payne, as is recorded in the Repertories and Journals of the City of London (13 and 15 Hustings Roll 251. Nos. 10. 11); and Richard Grafton, grocer, and the same Richard Payne, gentleman, were appointed trustees of the children of Thomas Berthelet, according to the then custom of the city.

CHAPTER III.

THE BOOKBINDINGS OF THOMAS BERTHELET, WITH DETAILED DESCRIPTIONS OF SOME TYPICAL EXAMPLES.

As has been shown, Thomas Berthelet lived in troublous times for bookbinding. He doubtless knew of the rich Mediæval bindings, which in his day were rapidly becoming scarce, and he was of course familiar with the old blind-stamped leather work as well as the brown panel stamps which were common at his time. He probably knew, also, the beautiful gold-tooled Italian bindings which came over from the Continent as rarities about the beginning of the sixteenth century. It will never be known with certainty whether Italian workmen came over here and taught Berthelet the art of gold-tooling on leather. If this was not the case, then Berthelet experimented for himself and soon became proficient, but several of his earlier bindings betray the hand of a tyro in this difficult art. In favour of the theory that an Italian gilder came to this country about the time that Berthelet became royal printer to Henry VIII. is the fact that there was at least one binding made for James V., King of Scotland, adorned with gold-tooling, executed on calf by some craftsman endowed with greater technical skill than Berthelet ever showed. This binding is, however, of a weaker design than Berthelet's are: his designs are never frittered as this one is; nevertheless, it must be noted that there are on the Scottish bindings some of the same stamps that Berthelet used, as well as others of a slighter and more ornate character. The volume is figured in the Dictionary of English Book Collectors, Part V., and in 1894 it belonged to the late Mr. Bernard Quaritch, of 15 Piccadilly, London.

Berthelet must have foreseen the very decorative possibilities that lay in the direction of gold-tooling on leather, promising indeed to compensate to a great extent for the loss of the beautiful and fast-disappearing Mediæval bindings in gold, silver, or ivory. He worked very energetically at his new art and quickly mastered it, the gilding on the majority of his books being excellent. His stamps were cut "solid," closely after Italian models, even if those he started with were not actually Italian stamps purchased by him from his problematical teacher. In time these designs became largely modified, but always retained much of the Italian feeling. Indeed, although Berthelet eventually developed a style of his own, the Italian inspiration is evident throughout. He could not have gone to a better school, as it is, with much justification, often held that the Italian gold-tooled bindings on leather of the late fifteenth and early sixteenth centuries are the finest in taste and altogether the most admirable ever produced. In consequence of the number of foreign books that came over here, it was incumbent on the native English workmen to do what they could to introduce a good style of indigenous work, and Berthelet was the most noted of the sixteenth-century binders who endeavoured to do this. The old English idea of the circle entered largely into his later and more ornamental designs, as also did the diamond, not in itself so original a style, as it frequently occurs elsewhere, amongst other places on books bound for Jean Grolier.

The bindings of the books printed by Thomas Berthelet have already in many instances been noticed as examples of fine workmanship, but he has not by any means always been credited with their authorship.

There are certain volumes which belonged to Henry VIII. at a period when Berthelet was royal printer, some of which were

PLATE XI.

VELVET BINDING OF A BIBLE PRINTED AT ZURICH IN
1543. MADE FOR HENRY VIII.

actually printed by him, on which certain stamps impressed in gold occur with great frequency. Several of these stamps are peculiar, and all of them bear the characteristics of being designed by the same artist, one who quite understood the art of designing curves for bookbindings. There is now little doubt that these bindings issued from Berthelet's workshop, and they may be safely considered to be his workmanship.

Unfortunately none of the bindings attributed to Berthelet are signed. There are numerous instances of signed bindings made in England both before and during his time, but these are always on panel stamps, which in all probability were seldom made by Englishmen. The fashion of signing a binding outside has indeed been seldom followed here, although it has been common on continental bindings for a long period. When English workmen have signed their bindings it has generally been by means of a small paper ticket pasted on the inside, or in very small letters or initials impressed at the lower edge of the inside of the boards.

Most of the bindings of the late fifteenth and early sixteenth centuries had silken ties fixed to the front edges of the boards. This peculiarity was probably a survival of an old custom which prevailed during the Middle Ages, when books were largely written on vellum, which is very apt to curl; the ties helped the thick, heavy boards to counteract this tendency. The ties on Berthelet's bindings are now nearly all rubbed off, but signs of them can be traced in most cases.

In default of a signed binding, we are driven, in Berthelet's case, to probability only with regard to fixing some standard by which to judge his work. The stamps used on all the books printed by Berthelet which are still in their original bindings are fortunately few in number, and nearly all these stamps are found on the first binding described in my list below. The gilding on this binding is bad, and evidently the work of a beginner, and I think it is the first English book ornamented with actual gold-tooling. It is dedicated to Henry VIII. and belonged to him, and my theory is, that the king desired Berthelet to try the new form of decoration on one of his own books, to be marked with his own heraldic devices and special royal badges. Berthelet doubtless considered the gold-tooling, which at that time he alone understood here, was a more distinguished manner of marking his work than the commoner plan of signing his name, as the foreign workmen were in the habit of doing on their large panel stamps.

The finest of Berthelet's bindings are all royal; those he made for private owners are rarely very highly ornamented. It is not known what kind of binding he executed before the time of his appointment as royal printer; indeed, it is quite possible that he did not begin binding until about that period; i. e., 1530. The chief official printing that he did was in the form of statutes, proclamations, single sheets, and other publications, which required no binding; but following the fashion of his time, when he did print an actual book, it is highly probable that he also bound it. The stamps he used on his earliest bindings were new to English work, and it seems probable that if they were not actually sent over to him from Italy he cut them closely resembling some Italian model. They were not used after his death, and this disuse of a binder's stamps after his own time is always something of a mystery. Stamps cut in metal for gilding designs on leather are very strong, and as the work they have to do is very light, they would, as a matter of fact, last much longer than they appear to if they were not destroyed purposely. Most great binders seem to have taken steps to insure the discontinuance of the use of their special stamps after their death, and so it is usually conceded that if the general design as well as the special stamps on any binding are similar to those found on any acknowledged work of a particular binder, this binding must then be his own work. Of course, other matters must be in proper accordance with such attribution,—leather, date, and heraldic marks, if any. Also in the case of a binder who produced much work, the fact of a binding having issued from his workshop would entitle it to be called his work, although his own hand may never have touched it.

The most important works in which figures and notices of Berthelet's bindings will be found are Mr. H. B. Wheatley's book on the "Remarkable Bindings in the British Museum," London, 1889, in which five specimens are figured in colour, none of them attributed to Berthelet, and they are all very bad plates; in Mr. R. R. Holmes's fine book on "Specimens of Royal Bookbinding from the Royal Library, Windsor Castle," London, 1893, in which two examples are figured, being fine plates in colour by Mr. Griggs, which two plates, with one other, are reproduced in the illustrated Catalogue of the Exhibition of Bookbindings held at the Burlington Fine Arts Club in 1891; Mr. W. Y. Fletcher's "English Bookbindings in the British Museum," London, 1895, in which several of Berthelet's finer bindings are naturally included, all shown in splendid colour plates by Mr. Griggs; and in my own monograph on "Royal English Bookbindings," published in 1896, in which there is one bad colour plate and one excellent half-tone (both by Evans) of acknowledged Berthelet bindings. Besides these few there are no good plates to be found; indeed, colour plates of bookbindings have been a source of much tribulation to authors until late years, when Mr. William Griggs, chromo-lithographer to the queen, has made a special study of their production, with the result that he can now produce the finest work of the kind to be found anywhere.

The immense majority of bookbindings made since the introduction of printing into England are in some sort of leather, and there is a very wide difference between the most elaborately decorated leather binding and the usual rich Mediæval bindings in precious metals, which they virtually superseded. In Berthelet's bill, quoted in the second chapter, will be found one or two entries which remind us that there really was a sort of connecting link between these two widely divergent schools of book decoration. This link is to be found in the embroidered bindings, some of which, in all probability bound by Berthelet, still remain. These bindings, without being intrinsically valuable, are very ornamental indeed, and as far as appearance goes, they may well have given satisfaction even to the magnificent taste of Henry VIII., without adding to their beauty the strong temptation of being worth relegating to the melting-pot. In the bill already quoted we find entries of books bound in velvet and in satin, and as a fact we also find among Henry VIII.'s books some which not only fit the descriptions to some extent, but having curves and designs upon them which, allowing for the unavoidable differences due to the material, strongly resemble some of Berthelet's curves as used on leather. The velvet bindings, some of which remain that belonged to Henry VII., also take their place as very decorative work; these are adorned in many cases with enamels, a form of ornamentation having, in common with embroidery, a strong claim to preservation because of its beauty, although equally of no intrinsic value. There is nothing to connect these earlier bindings with Berthelet. The one or two embroidered bindings which I venture to attribute to him, and describe below in their chronological order, have certainly in two instances some evidence to that effect inherent in themselves, inasmuch as they have on their edges Berthelet's usual legend painted in gold.

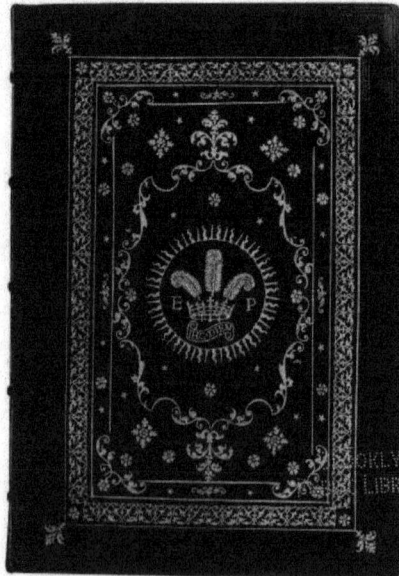

PLATE XII.

CALF BINDING OF "TROGUS POMPEIUS.
CHOROGRAPHICA, 1546" MADE FOR PRINCE EDWARD.

There are other embroidered books of the time of Henry VIII., which were worked for him by his daughter Elizabeth, but although these probably enough were put together for her by Berthelet, the designs upon them have nothing of his about them, having in all probability been designed by the princess herself. Some of these are at the Bodleian Library at Oxford, and others in the British Museum; the finest of them have been already figured and described.[A]

[A] Davenport, "English Embroidered Bookbindings." Kegan Paul, London, 1899.

There certainly are enough specimens left of such ornamental bindings to show that plain leather bindings were not always considered elaborate enough in appearance to compensate entirely for the loss of the gold-jewelled and enamelled productions which immediately preceded them; and it seems wonderful that bindings made in such apparently fragile materials as velvet and satin should not only be in existence but actually in a very good state of preservation, though faded in colour. They are really much more enduring than is generally imagined, but unquestionably numbers of them, worked on velvet, satin, and canvas, have perished or been worn out long ago. Embroidered books were made for all the Tudors, mostly on velvet, and a little later, in the time of Charles I., numbers of them, usually small, were embroidered on satin. The dates of the manuscripts bound in embroidered velvet and satin by Berthelet are not quite certain, but it is probable that his work of this kind in both these materials is the earliest made in England.

The greater number of bindings made by Thomas Berthelet belonged, as might be expected, to Henry VIII., Edward VI., or Mary; that is to say, they formed part of the old Royal Library of England. This old Royal Library, or as much as was then left of it, was given by George II. to the British Museum in 1757, and it forms perhaps the most valued special collection in that institution. It must not, however, be supposed that every old English royal book was really included in this library, for by some means or other a very considerable number of them were separated from the rest, and now exist scattered all over England, in private libraries as well as at Windsor. Such books now seldom come into the open market, and if they do, they are generally purchased by the state, and so return to their old companions. Also, royal bookbinders did some work outside their official limits, and small bindings of an unimportant kind, evidently the work of Berthelet, are not uncommon in England. They are always charming, and the simplicity of the quiet blind lines running side by side with others in bright gold on the rich brown calf is quite delightful; such simple covers usually have a rectangular panel with small Italian fleurons at the outer corners, and usually an initial, monogram, or heraldic ornament in the centre.

Before printing was used in England, the commonest leather for bindings was goat or sheep, but Berthelet found his favourite Italian bindings were largely bound in calf, a leather having a beautiful surface, and in some ways easier to gild than goat. I believe he was the first English binder to use this leather exclusively; it was rarely used in England before his time, although it was common on the Continent. His calf bindings, with few exceptions, are still in excellent condition, and are always of a beautiful rich brown colour. Many of these volumes have been, I think unnecessarily, rebacked; certainly in all such cases the old backs should have been preserved, which has not always been done. There is, however, no doubt that the calf used on Berthelet's bindings may still be considered quite sound, whereas books bound in that leather within the last fifty years, or even less, are now all powdering away. In spite of greater chemical knowledge and presumably better processes of tanning and preparing leather, the conclusion that this material, as produced to-day, is not a fitting one for books is forced upon us.

Berthelet used also a very decorative white leather, supposed to be deerskin or doeskin, prepared with lime in the same manner as vellum. This leather is soft and creamy in colour; it has a smooth surface and takes gilding to perfection. There are not many instances of its use, but those that do exist are always perfectly strong and sound, except where they show signs of fair wear and tear. The taste for white gilded leather began with Berthelet, and it has been highly esteemed as a style in England almost ever since. Such work was done for all our Tudor sovereigns, but the white deerskin soon gave place to vellum, especially during the time of our Stuart kings; and this, to some extent, has been used to the present day. Probably the strongest and most durable materials used for bookbinding at any time have been the white deerskin, white vellum, and white pigskin, the first two mentioned being chiefly used in England, and the last in Germany. This durability is most likely due to the method of preparation and the absence of any dye. Bark-tanned goatskin is also an excellent leather, and was much used in England from the twelfth century onwards.

Several of Berthelet's bindings bear legends, and texts, dates, and names, on their sides. These inscriptions are variously arranged, but as a rule they are contained in small long panels, sometimes in circles, and rarely simply impressed on the side of the book as its chief ornament. In the cases where coats of arms are given, the initials of the owner are generally added as well. The lettering on the sides of the books is either in Greek, Latin, French, or English, examples of each of which are described below, and there is never any lettering on the backs of any of them.

Except in so far as the wording of these inscriptions is concerned, which often reads consecutively on both sides, the ornamentation is alike on both boards of all Berthelet's bindings. The fondness for lettering sentences on the outside of his books did not stop, however, at the binding, as Berthelet carried it out also in several instances on the edges of the leaves themselves. The edges of these leaves were usually made a creamy colour, and a legend was painted upon them with gold paint. This legend, "Rex in Aeternum Vive," is a quotation from the Book of Daniel; it is sometimes followed by the mysterious word "Neez" or "Nez," which Mr. Edward Scott of the British Museum considers to be the three first letters of the words, Ναβουχοδονοσωρ Εσαει Ζηθι, as the phrase was addressed to that king. Whenever this legend is found on a decorative binding of the time of Henry VIII., I should say it is a sure sign of Berthelet's royal work.

Fortunately this legend, on some of Berthelet's earliest bindings, is associated with certain stamps of marked character, which can thus be safely considered his, and which enable us, even when they are found on other bindings without the legend, to attribute the work with certainty to him. It is my opinion that all the existing bindings in calf or white deerskin that were made for Henry VIII. and Edward VI., as well as most of those for Queen Mary, were Berthelet's work.

The legend on the edges of the leaves of some of Berthelet's books was not, however, the only way in which he decorated them. There are other instances where the whole edge is painted with heraldic designs in colour. This fore-edge decoration was not a new thing even in Berthelet's time, but he seems to have been the first to adopt it in England. To some extent the ornamentation of the edges of rare volumes has been practised ever since, both in this country and abroad. The most elaborate work of the kind was, I believe, from the hand of Samuel Mearne, royal binder to Charles II., and about a hundred years after his time the fashion was revived by James Edwards of Halifax. Both these binders painted the edges of their books so that the pictures showed only when held in a certain position. Possibly the lettering on the edges of some of Berthelet's books may have been suggested to him by the fact that in Mediæval times, when books were large and were kept on their sides with the front edges forward, it was no uncommon thing to write the title on these edges in large letters.

This title lettering is, however, very rarely ornamentally treated; it is only used as an eminently useful expedient. Berthelet makes it a decorative feature, and substitutes a legend, which may be considered as a sign of royal ownership, for the more usual title of the book.

From such collections and libraries in England as have been available to me I have chosen a few typical examples of Berthelet's work for detailed description. I have illustrated as many as possible of the finest specimens in colour plates by Mr. William Griggs, to whom my best thanks are due for the patience with which he has endured my superintendence of his work, and my compliments for the admirable results of his unequalled skill in this particular branch of colour-printing. Each of these colour plates must yet be a little discounted as to the apparent freshness of their appearance. I think that in all prints and photographs old objects gain in this way; nevertheless, most of the books illustrated are really wonderfully preserved. The half-tone and process blocks are also by Mr. Griggs, some of them from my own drawings; the methods of producing tone blocks capable of being printed with type have made great advances in late years, but I feel that in America better results are obtained in this particular branch of art than as yet can be made by English workmen. I have arranged the bindings which I have chosen for detailed descriptions in chronological order, taking the printed date as correct; it may not be actually so in all cases, but under the circumstances I think these dates are probably near enough for all present purposes.

1528-1530 (?). Galteri Deloeni Libellus de tribus Hierarchiis. MS. Dedicated to Henry VIII. Bound in brown calf, and tooled in gold with a few blind lines. The ornamentation consists in a filling in the spaces, mostly triangular, left by the intersections of a parallelogram aligned with the edges of the boards, and a diamond. In the centre is the royal coat of arms, crowned, cleverly outlined by reversed curves. Between the crown and the top of the shield are two double roses; above the crown are two stars; at the sides are two cornucopias. Below the shield are arabesques; four single daisies, the daisy being a badge used by Henry VIII. and Edward VI. in remembrance of their descent from Margaret of Beaufort; four stars, and stamps representing the crucifixion, and a serpent, with references to texts. The four large triangular spaces between the rectangle and the diamond are ornamented with arabesques, the upper and lower spaces bearing also a stamp of the single daisy. Beyond the diamond come the four large corners, each of which is decorated in a similar way. This binding is a remarkable one, inasmuch as it contains nearly all the small stamps that Berthelet subsequently used in so many combinations, and it is probably the earliest example of gold-tooling on an English leather binding. The gilding is not well executed, and it is likely enough that this is one of his first finished attempts at such work. It is rougher than any other example, but in spite of that it is very effective and rich in appearance.

Vitae illustrium Virorum. MS. Bound in brown calf, and gold-tooled with a few lines in blind, and measuring 14½ by 9½ inches.

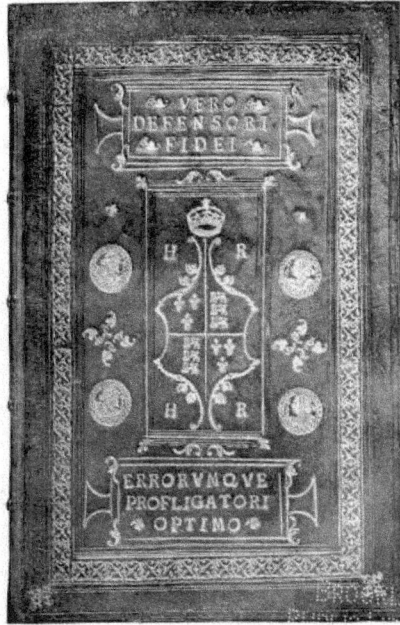

PLATE XIII.

CALF BINDING OF A MS. COMMENTARY ON THE
CAMPAIGN OF THE EMPEROR CHARLES V. AGAINST THE
FRENCH IN 1544. MADE FOR HENRY VIII., TO WHOM THE
MS. IS ADDRESSED.

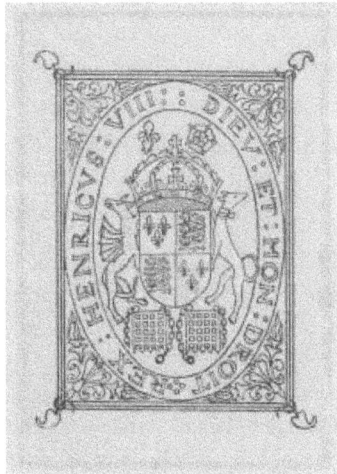

About 1528 Henry VIII. made a change in the supporters of his royal shield.
His father, Henry VII., who was very proud of his descent from Cadwallader,

the last of the British kings, adopted and used as one of his supporters the red dragon which had been a badge of that king. The red dragon was used by both Henry VII. and Henry VIII. as their dexter supporter, and with it, as a sinister supporter, they both also used the white greyhound. In or about 1528 Henry VIII. adopted a crowned lion statant as his dexter supporter, transferring the dragon to the sinister side, and leaving out the greyhound altogether. This lion still remains the dexter supporter of the royal coat of arms of England, but the dragon was discontinued on the accession of James I. to the throne of England, a unicorn, one of the supporters of the ancient Scottish coat of arms, being substituted for it. So that the stamp which forms the principal ornament on this book was probably cut about 1528, certainly not much later; indeed, it is possible that this was one of the books bound by Berthelet for the king before his appointment as royal printer. The coat of arms is contained within an oval ribbon bearing the words, "REX HENRICVS VIII. DIEV ET MON DROIT." The coat is ensigned with a large royal crown, has a dragon supporter on the dexter side and a greyhound on the sinister; above the crown is a fleur-de-lys and a double rose, and two portcullises depend by chains from the lower edge of the shield. The oval is contained within a close rectangular panel, the inner angles of which are filled with an arabesque design. At each outer corner is a leaf of Venetian character.

Above and below the rectangle is a crowned double rose, flanked by the letters K H,—mysterious letters, the meaning of which is not yet understood. Beyond this again comes a broad double border of a narrow running pattern containing a fleur-de-lys and a triple floral ornament. This same border occurs on several of Berthelet's earlier bindings. The inner corners of the rectangular border are filled with a symmetrical design of a vase with flowers and two curves terminating in human masks. There were originally some outer lines of small gold-tooling, but these, as well as the corners, have been "repaired" away.

On a fly-leaf in this volume is a note which says: "Codex hic fuit olim Henrici VIII., ei Jo. Leylandus Titulum fecit—Vitae illustrium virorum, etc." John Leyland, the antiquary, was keeper of the king's library about 1530.

This book undoubtedly should be with the rest of the old royal library at the British Museum, and its inclusion among the books at Oxford is explained by the Rev. W. Dunn Macray in his book, "The Annals of the Bodleian Library," in which he mentions the interesting fact that in August, 1605, King James I. visited the Bodleian and offered to present to Sir T. Bodley, "from all the libraries of the royal palaces, whatever precious and rare books he might choose to carry away." So that, in fact, instead of feeling that we in London should have the few "outside" royal books returned to us, we should perhaps feel a debt of gratitude to Sir T. Bodley for leaving anything at all in the libraries of the royal palaces, in face of King James's generous offer.

1530 (?). The third volume of a copy of the Works of St. Chrysostom, printed at Basle in 1530, has very kindly been shown to me by Mr. E. Gordon Duff, librarian of the Ryland's Library, Manchester. It is bound in calf, and one side is almost completely destroyed, but the other is in a fairly good condition. It measures 15 by 10 inches, is tooled with gold and blind lines, and bears as a centre ornament a rectangular panel with the royal coat of arms of Henry VIII. ensigned with a large crown, having as a dexter supporter a greyhound and on the sinister side a dragon. This arrangement of the supporters is wrong, but it is possibly unintentional, and due to the forgetfulness of the engraver when he drew the design on his metal plate. Above the crown are two double roses, and above it are scattered impressions of a ring with a dot in the middle. Below the shield are two portcullises, chained, with a few tufts of grass. This handsome coat of arms is enclosed by a border on which are the words, "DIEV ET MON DROIT," and small stamps of a leaf, a single rose, and a fleur-de-lys; above and below are impressions of a stamp of a large double rose, crowned, flanked by the letters K H. These initials are somewhat of a puzzle. They have been interpreted as simply meaning King Henry, and perhaps this solution is the easiest way out of the difficulty; but it is not altogether satisfactory. Besides "King," the only other word for which the letter K is likely to stand is the name "Katherine," and it could only then have stood for either Katharine of Aragon, who was divorced in 1533; Katherine Howard, who was married in 1540 and was beheaded in 1543; or Katharine Parr, who was married in 1543 and survived the king.

A very decided objection to the theory that the initial K belonged to any of these queens is found in the fact that it precedes that of the king himself, which is not at all likely to have occurred under the circumstances. In the volume to be described presently, where the initials H A are presumed to be those of "Henry" and "Anne," an example is found of the more likely way in which such initials would occur.

The inner panel is enclosed, at a considerable distance, by a broad triple border, and the inner corners of this border are curiously ornamented with ornamental gold-tooling arranged in quarter-circle form. This style of corner ornamentation was common in Italy, but very rare in England, at the time this book was made. The inner angles of each quarter-circle bear triple impressions from a stamp of trefoil shape bearing small scroll-work of Oriental character upon it, the ground gold and the design showing in the leather. The segments of circles beyond this inner angle are ornamented consecutively with a row of fleur-de-lys and single roses alternately; a row of small long-shaped knots, often found on Italian books, and also occurring on one bound for King James V. of Scotland; a row of wavy flames; and beyond all, in the center of the quarter-circle, impressions in gold of a leaf with stalk flanked by two roses.

These corners, as well as the inner rectangular panel and the inner line of the outer panel, are all marked by lines of blind-tooling, which are mitred at the corners.

The outer border consists of an inner line of wavy flames, a broadish line of circles crossed with arabesques, and an outer line of numerous impressions from the small long-shaped knot stamp, and beyond all are a few blind lines.

This binding is in many ways a very remarkable one. The gold-tooling upon it is rough, but among the tools which are evidently Berthelet's are others which are not found on any other of his bindings. I think it is an early work, and that the existence upon it of the few delicate Italian stamps can be accounted for only by the theory that an Italian workman brought them over with him and taught Berthelet the art of gold-tooling. In the case of this particular volume, it is possible that it was one of those done by Berthelet under the eye of his master, and that he used some of his foreign tools as well as others belonging to himself.

Whatever may be the true explanation of these difficulties, there is no doubt that the binding is a most valuable and interesting one, and I thank Mr. E. Gordon Duff very sincerely for having allowed me to see it and to have it photographed for this monograph. The edges are gilded and ornamented with an arabesque design marked upon them by means of successive impressions from a small ring-shaped stamp.

The decoration of the corners of the boards of a binding with ornamentation arranged as a quarter-circle was very rare in England until the reign of Queen Elizabeth, at which time it was often found; then under the Stuart Kings James I. and Charles I. it probably reached its fullest development, and was especially favoured at Little Gidding. It is found on fifteenth-century Italian bindings, used with great skill, so that its occurrence on one of Berthelet's early bindings is not to be wondered at, the curious thing being rather that he did not use it more. As it now is, I think this book is the earliest existing English specimen of the use of this kind of ornamentation.

1530 (?). An interesting example in which the decoration of a binding is arranged with some reference to the contents of the book occurs on the cover of a French manuscript on "La Science de Geometrie," dedicated to King Henry VIII., and bound for him in white deerskin by Thomas Berthelet. This volume should always have been with the rest of the old Royal Library of England now in the British Museum, but by some means it became separated, and was recently purchased by the trustees of that institution from Mr. Cornish of Manchester.

The sides are ornamented with blind lines and gold-tooling; a large rectangular panel is marked out near the edges of the boards with fleurons at each outer corner; inside the panel near the top are the words, "VIVAT REX," in an ornamental cartouche of architectural elevation; below this, and filling up most of the remaining space, are three narrow elongated pyramids with triangular bases; the ground is dotted irregularly with small stars and dots. In the lower part of the panel is the word "GEOMETRIA" and a decorative scroll. This is the only instance I know in which the lettering outside any of Berthelet's bindings has any reference to the contents of the book.

On the white edges are the words, "REX IN AETERNVM VIVE NEZ," ornamentally written in gold in large capital letters.

1534. Bible, Antwerp, 1534. In two volumes. Bound in brown calf, tooled in blind and gold, and measuring 14½ by 9 inches. The design on each of these fine volumes is the same, but the lettering upon them is different. The words on volume I. are, "AINSI QUE TOUS MEURENT PAR ADAM—AVSSY TOVS SERONT VIVIFIES PAR CHRIST"; and on volume II., "LA LOY A ESTE DONNEE PAR MOYSE—LA GRACE ET LA VERITE EST FAICTE PAR JESU CHRIST." These words are in large gilt capitals in short lines, each word where necessary being divided from the next by a

PLATE XIV.

CALF BINDING OF "LA CYROPEDIE DE XENOPHON. PARIS, 1547." MADE FOR EDWARD VI.

small cross-crosslet. The lines are contained in a rectangular panel, with large corner stamps of a vase with flowers and two floral curves terminating in human masks. The triangular spaces thus left above and below the inscription are each filled by a double rose, crowned, flanked by the letters H A, perhaps standing for "Henry" and "Anne." Beyond the panel and touching it is a broad border, made up of a double line of stamps cut in the form of an ornamental fleur-de-lys and a three-lobed flower. Beyond the border is a space broken at the corner with a repetition of the vase stamp, enclosing which was in all probability a narrow fillet variously ornamented with small designs like that which occurs below the lettering on the second volume.

Both these volumes have been unfortunately restored in places, but the old patterns have to some extent been preserved, and new stamps cut on the lines of the old ones, as can be seen by reference to a binding now at Oxford which is treated in a very similar way, and which, although it also has received some attention from an inferior binder, has not been restored in a like disastrous manner.

1534. Opus de vera differentia regiae potestatis. Londini, T. Berthelet, 1534; measuring 8 by 5¼.

This volume is very like that at the Bodleian, already fully described on page 69. The centre stamp is the same, and so are the outer border and corners, but the handsome double border is wanting. The book has been badly repaired; in some cases stamps have been cut after the old patterns, but in others, as for instance the corners next to the oval label, they have been made in a modern arabesque pattern, not like the original. The book itself is a fine specimen of Berthelet's printing on vellum. The heraldic centre stamp, bearing the dragon and greyhound supporters, is really an anachronism; properly the supporters should be a lion and a dragon; the stamp, however, was seldom used, so Berthelet, having it by him, did not trouble to cut another, as he should have done.

1536. A charming little specimen of Berthelet's private binding is now in the Ryland's Library at Manchester, and by the courtesy of the librarian, Mr. E. Gordon Duff, I am enabled to describe it.

It is a remarkably fine copy of the New Testament, Tyndale's version, printed in London in 1536; there is an inscription inside which shows that in 1676 it belonged to Henry, Duke of Newcastle, and later to Dr. Charles Chauncey.

It is bound in brown calf, and has on each side a long upright panel within a border of ornamented circles of Italian design. The panel has on one side a unicorn in the centre, and on the other a talbot, the crest of the Heydon family. There are also some initials upon it, but these do not seem to throw any light upon its ownership. The badges are surrounded with scrolls made up of reversed curves, in Berthelet's usual manner. At the outer corners of the border are large Italianate fleurons, and the gold lines are supported by others in blind, running parallel to them. There are the remains of two silk ties.

1536. An historically interesting volume has just been bequeathed to the British Museum by the late Baron Ferdinand Rothschild, formerly member of Parliament for Waddesdon, who left altogether a very valuable collection of jewels and manuscripts to the British nation.

This volume is very large, measuring about 19¼ by 13½; it is a manuscript translation in French of the Decameron of Boccaccio, by Laurent de Premierfait, made from a Latin version by Antoine de Aresche, in 1414. The manuscript itself, which is illuminated, was probably made late in the fifteenth century.

The binding is in very dark calf, and is tooled in gold, with a few blind lines; it was made for Edward Seymour, first Duke of Somerset, the Protector, who was beheaded on Tower Hill in 1552.

The duke's motto, "FOY POVR DEBVOIR," is contained within an ornamental cartouche in the centre of each cover. The cartouche is enclosed, at some distance, in a diamond stamped with a small roll pattern; near each of the outer sides of the diamond is an ornament made of two impressions of a cornucopia stamp. Along the edges of the boards is a broad Italianate arabesque border; the inner angles of the border are filled with either the stamp of Plato or that of Dido, already described, enclosed in arabesques, and the outer corners have small fleurons.

The volume has been rebacked and some of the gold-tooling restored. The stamps found upon it are generally such as were used by Berthelet early in his career; but as there is no other indication of the date, it must be remembered that my attribution of the work as having been made about 1536 is only conjectural.

1538. Berthelet's "leather" curves turned into gold cord may be clearly seen on the red satin binding of a collection of sixteenth-century tracts bound probably about 1538. This curious volume is, as far as can be ascertained at present, the earliest English book bound in satin. It is very probably Berthelet's work,—indeed, it may actually be one referred to in the Letters and Papers of Henry VIII., Vol. 13, Part 2, p. 539, concerning which we are told that the king paid 6s. 8d. to "Bartlett the king's printer's servant that brought a book covered with crimosin saten embroidered." It measures 12 by 8 inches, and has been stupidly rebacked with leather, but is otherwise in good condition. There is an arabesque border parallel with the edges of the boards, made full at each of the four corners, and amplified across the centre into a kind of ornamental bridge. Not only are the curves and scrolls strongly suggestive of Berthelet's designs, but on the cream-coloured edges of the book are the words, "REX IN AETERNVM VIVE NEZ," which, as has already been remarked, may of itself be taken as an almost sure sign of Berthelet's work. Many of the scrolls are very similar to those which are used on a velvet binding described under the date 1543, which I think was also bound by Berthelet.

1540 (?). Jul. Claud Iguini oratio ad Hen. VIII. MS. This is bound in dark brown calf, and is ornamented very simply with gold-tooling and blind lines. In the centre is a well-designed stamp of the royal coat of arms, ensigned by a very large crown, and encircled by a garter with buckle, and bearing the motto, "Honi soit qui mal y pense." This design is enclosed between four Greek words, ΗΑΙΟΣ ΠΑΝΤΑΣ ΑΛΑΙΕΝΟΝ ΕΞΑΡΚΤΟΤ, the signification of which is not clear. A simple rectangular border in gold, made up of successive impressions of one of Berthelet's happily designed curves, completes a design which, although plain, is yet very charming.

1540. There is a fine specimen of one of Berthelet's bindings in white doeskin in the library of Trinity College, Oxford. It measures about 9 by 6 inches, and is a copy of "Theophylacti in omnes divi Pauli epistolas enarrationes, etc. Basileae, 1540." The sides are fully gilt, and ornamented with scroll-work and royal badges. In the centre is the crowned royal coat of arms of Henry VIII., surrounded by four chief decorative points, bearing, respectively, the royal initials, crowned, and crowned badges, double rose, fleur-de-lys, and portcullis. Each of these small designs is contained within a framework of golden scrolls, and the remaining space is rather closely filled with a rich tracery of scrolls and arabesques symmetrically arranged. The broad edges are cream coloured, and on them in large capitals are the words, "REX IN ETERNUM VIVE."

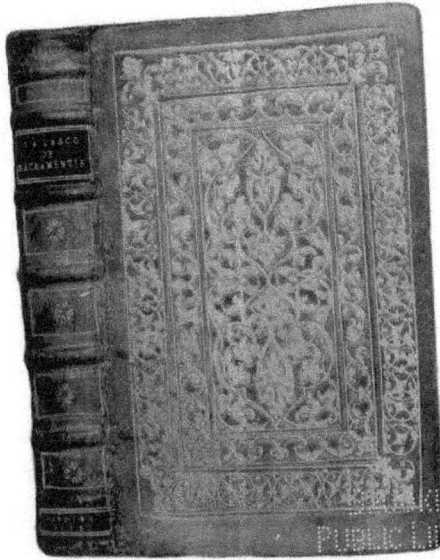

PLATE XV.

WHITE LEATHER BINDING OF "JOANNES A LASCO. BREVIS
DE SACRAMENTIS ECC. CHRISTI TRACTATIO. LONDON
1552."

1541. Elyot. The Image of Governance. T. Berthelet, London, 1541. Bound in white deerskin, and tooled in gold with a few blind lines. In the centre is an irregular panel made up with curves and arabesques, within which are the words, "DIEU ET MON DROIT." The panel is enclosed within an outer line of cleverly arranged scrolls, at the sides of which are the letters H R. An outer rectangular border of small S-shaped stamps, with fleurons at the outer corners, encloses the whole, the inner corners being filled with more scroll-work and arabesques. The ground is dotted with stamps of a daisy, a small circle stamp, and a five-pointed star.

A single daisy is impressed in gold in the centre of each of the panels on the back, and on the white edges of the book itself the words, "REX IN ETERNUM VIVE," are written in gold in capital letters.

1543. A Bible printed at Zurich in 1543, bound in orange-coloured velvet, which was probably originally some shade of crimson, is embroidered with designs outlined in gold cord. It measures 15 by 9¼ inches, and has been ruinously rebacked with leather. It forms part of the old English Royal Library at the British Museum, and belonged to King Henry VIII.

The king's initials, tied together by a knot, are in the centre, within a circle, above and below which are symmetrical curves of like character to those on several of Berthelet's leather bindings, from which no doubt these are taken. A broad rectangular border encloses the central panel, and is ornamented with large double Tudor roses at each corner, the rest of the border space being cleverly filled with repetitions, right and left, of a simple fleuron with leaves.

The central circle, as well as the forms of the scrolls used in this binding, are all suggestive of Berthelet's methods of design; and in consideration of the fact that he actually mentions velvet books in his bill as having been bound by himself (p. 43), I think that this binding may be claimed as his with some degree of probability. If the designs were on leather, one or other of Berthelet's known stamps would fit them all. Several of the curves are very similar to those worked on the satin bindings of 1536, already described. The edges of the leaves are elaborately painted in colour, the groundwork being creamy white; on the upper edge at the top is a winged cherub, in the centre is a large gold fleur-de-lys on a blue ground, enclosed in a red eight-pointed framework, and beneath this is a square panel in which is a flying dove; the remainder of the space is filled with graceful arabesques, with figures and fleurons in gold and colour. The front edge is not in good condition, as it naturally has been more affected by use, and some of the painting is obliterated. It is ornamented with five principal designs, all of which are connected by an ornamental framework,—scrolls, flowers, and arabesques in gold and colour. The five designs, beginning at the top, are: a small rectangular cartouche with a figure of God the Father; the royal coat of arms, crowned, within a laurel wreath tied with white ribbon; a broad oblong of dark colour, on which was most probably the word "BIBLIA" in gold; a large red rose with white centre within a circle; and a small rectangular panel, the design upon which has been worn off. The lower edge, at the bottom of the book, has nearest the back a satyr upholding scrolls, in the middle a circle, the design upon which has been obliterated by wear, and near the front edge an arabesque pattern.

This is the most highly decorative book edge which exists on any English book of the early sixteenth century, and when it was first done must have attracted much attention and admiration, as it is excellently painted. There is hand-painting in colour inside the book, especially on the title-page, and it is very probable that the same artist executed all this work, both inside and outside, as there is a great similarity of style.

1546. In Trogum Pompeivm sive Ivstinvm chorographica ad excellentiss. Dominum D. Edwardvm Principem, etc., 1546. A manuscript list of countries and cities mentioned in Trogus Pompeius and in the Epistles of Cicero, addressed to Prince Edward by Petrus Olivarius.

Bound in brown calf, rather lighter than usual, measuring 10¼ by 7¼ inches, and bearing in the centre the badge of three ostrich feathers within a prince's coronet, with a label bearing the words, "IHC DIEN," and flanked by the initials E P.

Prince Edward never was Prince of Wales, a title which is conferred on the eldest son only at the pleasure of the sovereign. The triple-feather badge, which certainly has been associated with this title ever since Edward VI., and has been used as a special badge by all the Princes of Wales since his time, is, however, originally not connected especially with Wales or with any particular son of the sovereign. It was first used by the descendants of Edward III., and appears to have been considered a family badge, borne by them because of their ancestress, Queen Philippa of Hainault. The feathers were the cognizance of the Province of Ostrevant, an appanage of the eldest sons of the House of Hainault. The motto, "IHC DIEN," seems really to have been used by the Blind King of Bohemia, who was killed at Crecy, and the Black Prince adopted it as his own; the two have been inseparable ever since.

On this binding the ostrich plume and its belongings are enclosed within a circle of flames, alternately straight and wavy; the circle is within an oval cleverly marked by a succession of curved arabesques, in the designing of which Berthelet was very skilled, several of them being capable of effective and even surprising combinations. They have something of the quality so valued by designers of wall-papers, and fit each other in a very remarkable way. The ground is ornamentally dotted with roses, stars, and a diamond-shaped floral ornament. The arabesque oval has a handsome symmetrical fleuron at the top and bottom, and is enclosed within a rectangular border of rather elaborate design. First is a gold line with ornamental corners; within it is another gold line, the intermediate space being dotted with small arabesques, single roses, and five-pointed stars; then comes a richly designed Italianate fillet with roses at each outer corner, and an outer line with fleurons at each of the outer corners. The book is divided into four panels. As is usual on all Berthelet's bindings in calf, there are a few blind lines as well.

1544. A Commentary in Latin on the Campaign of the Emperor Charles V. against the French in 1544, addressed by Antonius de Musica to Henry VIII.; in manuscript; measures 12¼ by 8¼ inches.

It is bound in deep brown calf, and tooled in gold with some lines in blind. In the centre, within an upright panel of gold and blind lines with small fleurs-de-lys at the corners, is the royal coat of arms of Henry VIII., cleverly outlined with reversed curves, crowned, and flanked with the letters H R, repeated twice. Directly above and below the central panel are two broad rectangular cartouches made in gold lines, and small arabesques with "anvil" handles. In each of these cartouches is a legend; those on the upper cover contain the words, "VERO DEFENSORI FIDEI | ERRORVMQVE PROFLIGATORI OPTIMO"; those on the lower cover, "MAXIMO HENRICO OCTAVO | REGI ANGLORVM FRANC. HIBERNIEQVE, P. M. P. P. D. G." No one has yet elucidated the signification of these last letters. The centre panel is flanked on

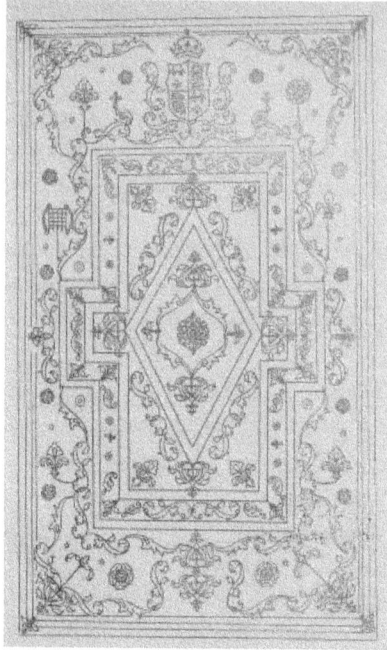

PLATE XVI.

WHITE LEATHER BINDING OF "D. AURELII AUGUSTINI HIPPONENSIS EP. TAM IN VETUS QUAM IN NOVUM TEST. COMMENTARII. BAS., 1542." MADE FOR QUEEN MARY.

one side by two impressions of a portrait stamp of Plato, and on the other two of Dido, the remaining spaces being sparsely filled with leaf stamps. An outer border of Italian design, with fleurons at each outer corner, encloses the whole. The small medallion stamps containing portraits of Dido and Plato, which are found on this volume, were often used by Berthelet as the chief ornamentation on small books bound by him. They usually occur singly as a centre ornament within a gold line panel, with small fleurons at the outer corners.

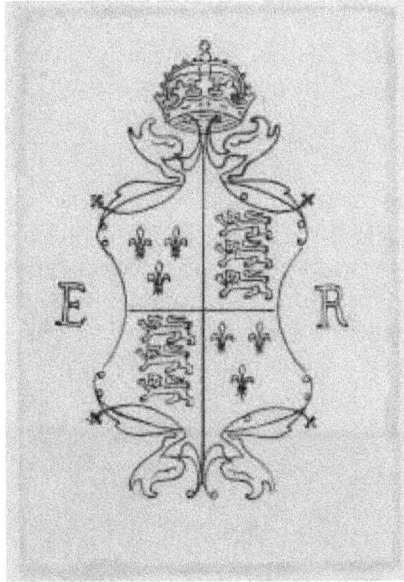

1547. Xenophon. La Cyropedie. Paris 1547.

Bound in rich brown calf, and ornamented with gold-tooling, black fillets, and some blind lines. In the centre is the royal coat of arms of Edward VI., very effectively outlined with arabesques, crowned, and flanked by the letters E R. Above and below the coat is a double rose and two five-pointed stars.

The royal shield is contained within two interlaced fillets, outlined in gold and stained black; the inner is in the shape of an upright diamond; the outer is turned and curved upon itself so as to make a double border. The spaces left between these various curves and lines are filled with gold ornaments, the most noticeable of which is a large stamp of a cornucopia. The other small stamps are arabesques and five-pointed stars. The outer corners are marked by a gilt fleuron, and on the front edge of each board are the remains of two ties. The back probably had double roses stamped in gold between each of the bands, but the book, which is, with this exception, in excellent condition, has recently been restored here with new stamps cut after the old pattern.

1547 (?). In the Advocates' Library at Edinburgh is a fine specimen of Berthelet's work in binding. It was bound for Edward VI. in calf, and bears in the centre his coat of arms flanked by the initials E R, and above and below the coat, on each side, is a long rectangular panel with a kind of handle at each end, like those found afterwards on the horn-books. The legends on the panels read, on the upper cover, "An idle or deceitful hande maketh pore | But a diligent Labourynge hand maketh ryche. Proverb. 10"; and on the under cover, "No man lyghteth a candle and putteth it | in a privie place—neither under a bushell. Luke II." In the panels of the back are, alternately, a small upright lion and a fleur-de-lys.

1548. Among the books bound by Berthelet for King Edward VI. is a small copy of Ptolemy's *Geografia*, printed at Venice in 1548. It is simply bound in calf, with a plain gilt line along the edges of the boards, and the words, "Omnis potestas a Deo," in a cartouche in the middle of the side. As far as the binding goes, this volume is one of Berthelet's simplest, and I should not, for that reason, have noticed it here; but the book is remarkable because of the way he has painted the edges. These are pale blue, and are ornamented with heraldic designs on shields. On the upper edge is

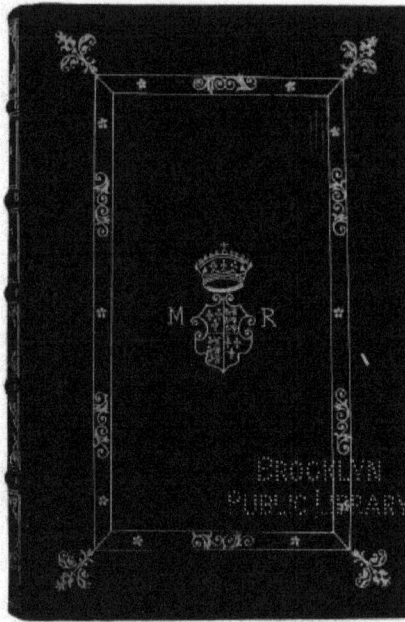

PLATE XVII.

CALF BINDING OF QUEEN MARY'S PRAYER BOOK. MS. ON
VELLUM. BOUND FOR THE QUEEN.

the coat of arms of France, on the front edge that of England, and on the lower that of Ireland. These shields are flanked by the initials of the king, and the rest of the space is filled with a very prettily arranged interlaced strapwork in black, in and out of which wind delicate, graceful curves and flowers painted in gold.

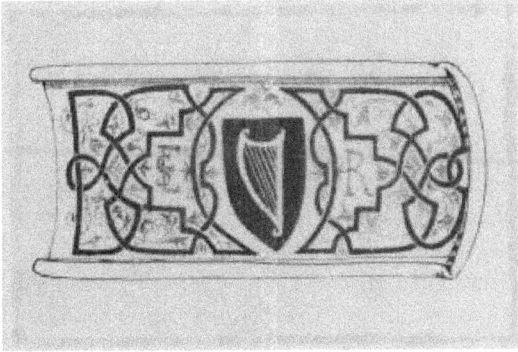

1548. Bude. Commentarii linguae Graecae, etc. Parisiis, 1548. 13-3/4 by 9.

Bound in brown calf, and ornamented with gold-tooling and some blind lines. In the centre the royal coat of arms of Edward VI., crowned, is flanked by the letters E R, above and below each of which is a small five-petalled flower. The coat is enclosed between two interlaced squares, outlined in gold and stained black. At each of the four corners of the horizontal square is a floral arabesque in gold, with a spray of pear.

The centre design is enclosed at a considerable distance by a broad black fillet, outlined in gold, parallel to the edges of the board, mitred in gold at the corners, and decorated alternately at short intervals along its length with scrolls and small five-petalled flowers stamped in gold. The inner angles of the fillet are marked by a gold double rose, and the outer angles by an elaborate fleuron in outline.

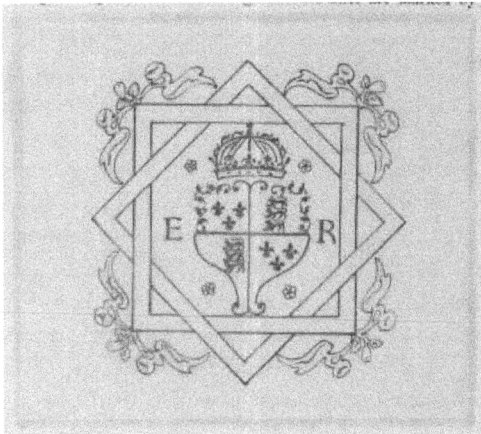

1550. Andreasius. De amplitudine misericordiae Dei, etc. Basileae, 1550; measures 6 by 4 inches. It is bound in rich brown calf, the royal coat of arms of Edward VI. being placed in the centre, flanked by the letters E R. Parallel with the edges of the boards are lines in gold and blind, with small fleurs-de-lys in gold at the four inner corners and arabesque fleurons at the outer corners. Although this little book is very simple, it is nevertheless very charming, the beautiful brown colour of the calf being well brought out by the bright gold lines and the dark blind lines.

1552. Bembo. Historiae Venetae. Lib. XII. Venetiis, 1551; measures 12 by 9 inches. It is bound in brown calf, and ornamented with gold-tooling, blind lines, and black fillets. In the centre is the royal coat of arms of Edward VI., to whom the book belonged, enclosed in a very cleverly interwoven fillet outlined in gold and stained black. This fillet is so arranged in straight and curved pieces as to give the general effect of being arranged in eight circles and eight semicircles. The coat of arms, ensigned with the royal crown, is outlined by arabesques and surrounded by ten small stars, six of which are within a single curved-line border having fleurons and daisies at its four extremities, and four without it, beyond which comes the inner broken line of the fillet, spreading out at the top into a large circle, within which are the words, "DIEV ET MON DROYT," and below into another circle, also large, bearing the date MDLII. Flanking the coat of arms are two small circles, within which are the crowned initials E R. The fillet now takes a rectangular form, and extends upwards and downwards from these small circles, while the irregular corner spaces left between this rectangle and the outer edges of the inner line of the fillet are each ornamented with one handsome reversed arabesque, with fleuron, two stars, and a double daisy. Four large circles of equal size to that enclosing the royal motto are arranged over the right-angled corners of the mitred parallelogram which is part of the fillet, and the spaces within these circles are each filled with an ornament made up of a graceful reversed arabesque, with a fleuron and three small flowers. Where the fillet becomes the outer border of the design it is rectangular in form, broken by semicircular indentations in the centre of each of the four sides; in these hollows are arabesques and double daisies. The remaining spaces just within the outer border are filled, top and bottom, with short lines of the cornucopia stamp, with double daisies and stars, and at each side by an impression of a handsome arabesque curve with one small flower. At each of the outer corners is a double daisy. As a book this is a curious specimen, the back being arranged and gilded so as to resemble the front, and unless the volume is carefully examined it appears to have no back at all. This is the earliest instance of this peculiarity known to me, but I have met with a few similar cases of later date and in Italian work. It has nothing to recommend it, and is useless and ugly as well as being constructively vicious. It is interesting to note that Berthelet here reverts, perhaps unknowingly, to the old English appreciation of the decorative use of the circle. This is probably, in all details, the finest binding he ever made.

1552. Joannes a Lasco. Brevis de Sacramentis Ecclesiae Christi Tractatio, etc. London, 1552; measures 5½ by 3½ inches, and is bound in cream-coloured deer or doe skin and tooled in gold. There are two holes for tie-ribbons near the front edge of each board.

The decoration consists of a central rectangular panel closely filled with solid arabesques symmetrically arranged. The panel is enclosed in a double border, the inner division of which has an arabesque filling and small fleurons at each angle; the outer is ornamented with repetitions of a circular stamp intersected by arabesque forms of a pattern very commonly found on Berthelet's work, and closely copied from an Italian original; at each of the angles is a large fleuron. The narrow space between the edge of the boards and the outer border is ornamented with scattered impressions of a small crescent and a diamond.

Each of the panels of the back contains a single impression from a small four-petalled flower stamp. The edges of the leaves are gilded, and upon them is a wavy spray of vine, with leaves and grape clusters, impressed by means of a small ring stamp.

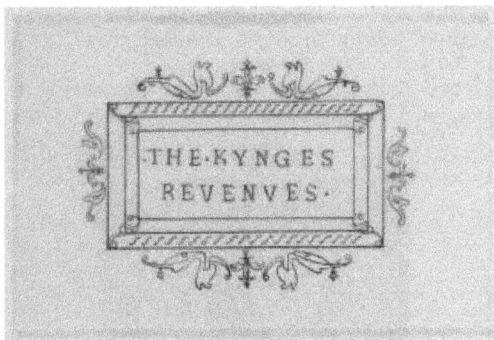

1552. The King's Revenues. The original certificate of the state of the revenues of King Edward VI., drawn up on the 10th of Decr. 1552, by Thomas Lord Darcy, Thomas (Thirlby), Bishop of Norwich, Sir Richard Cotton, Sir John Gate, Sir Robert Bowes, and Sir Walter Mildmay, His Majesty's Commissioners. With their signatures appended. MS. on vellum, measuring 15-3/4 by 11 inches.

Bound in brown calf, tooled in blind and gold. In the centre is the royal coat of arms of England flanked by the letters E R, and crowned. The outline of the shield is skilfully made by impressions from the pair of arabesque stamps used in the ornamentation of the two decorative rectangular cartouches above and below it. On the upper of these small panels are lettered the words, "THE KYNGES REVENVES," and on the lower, "Anno quinto Regis Edwardi Sexti"; and they are further adorned with "solid" stamps in gold of an Italian character. The border has a handsome gilt-tooled design enclosed within eight lines in blind; the pattern of the gilt part is taken from an Italian model. There are gilt fleurons at the outer and inner corners of the panel.

1553. Strena Galteri Deloeni, ex Capite Geneseos quarto deprompta, etc. MS. Dedicated to Edward VI., and measuring 5-3/4 by 4 inches.

Bound in cream-coloured deerskin and tooled in blind and gilt. In the centre is the royal coat of arms flanked by the initials E R, and surmounted by a double rose, above which is a royal crown. Just below the coat of arms is another stamp of the double rose. Above and below each of the initial letters is a very graceful stamp of a cornucopia. The upper part of the panel is filled with stamps of two arabesque scrolls, two double roses, and a daisy; the lower part has two double roses, and a daisy with stalk and two leaves. The inner corners of the panel are marked with long stems, at the end of each of which is a small fleuron, and the remaining spaces are dotted freely with a small six-rayed star. All these stamps are found constantly on Berthelet's bindings.

This is the only book bound in white deerskin for Edward VI. at present known.

1553. D. Aurelii Augustini Hipponensis episcopi, tam in vetus quam in nouum Testamentum Commentarij, etc. Basileae, 1542.

Bound in white deerskin for Queen Mary, and measuring 12¼ by 8 inches. The coat of arms on this volume is put in a very unusual

PLATE XVIII.

CALF BINDING OF "EPITOME OMNIUM OPERUM DIVI AURELII AUGISTINI. COL., 1549." MADE FOR QUEEN MARY.

place. It is near the top of the design, the centre ornament being merely an arabesque. The boards have an irregular rectangular double-lined panel with right-angled projections at each side, outlined in gold; within these lines are small fleurons at the angles, and small scrolls, fleurs-de-lys, and rosettes. Between the centre and the inner edge of the plain panel is a double-lined diamond, edged with curves and scrolls, the corners ornamented with fleurons. Between the outer edge of the panel and the edge of the book are curves and Tudor badges, each held up either by a curved or a straight stalk, the royal coat of arms forming the chief ornament at the top, and two double roses at the bottom. The corners are closely and cleverly filled with a few curves reversed again and again. The original book is in a perfectly sound state, but the gilding upon it became rubbed, and many years ago it fell into the hands of an unscrupulous restorer, who regilded it all over with stamps cut to some extent like the old ones, but not exactly. The impressions of the old stamps still remain quite sufficiently to be recognized, and I have made a drawing of this binding, which shows the original form of its decoration. It is one of the latest bindings made by Berthelet, and in some ways it must have been one of his finest.

However much it may be considered advisable or necessary to replace old leather on bindings by new, it is quite certain that no state of decay can under any circumstances justify the regilding or restamping of any gold-tooled work. This unfortunately has been a favourite proceeding with many binders, with disastrous effects, and it cannot be too strongly condemned from every point of view.

1553 (?). A manuscript poem of controversy against the Reformers is addressed to Queen Mary by Myles Haggard; bound in calf, and tooled in gold and blind, by Berthelet. It measures about 9 by 6 inches, and has the remains of green silk ties on the front edges of the boards. In the centre is the royal coat of arms, crowned, and flanked by two scrolls, all contained within a circle stained black and outlined with gold lines, the outer edge being ornamented with a series of impressions of a small flame-shaped stamp on a narrow, slightly curved foot. The initials of Queen Mary, M R, are shown twice, arranged squarely, just beyond the flamed circle.

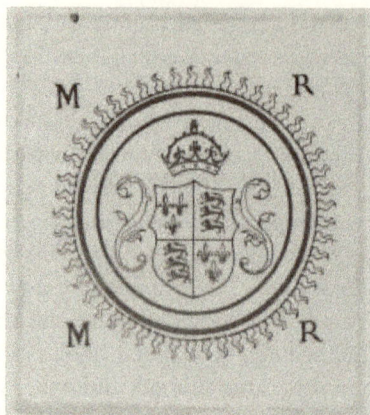

There is a gold line, with blind, parallel and near to the edges of the boards, and at the outer angles of this rectangle are arabesque fleurons. In the panels of the back are single impressions of small roses.

1554 (?). Horae Beatae Mariae Virginis, etc., or Queen Mary's Prayer-Book, written on vellum and beautifully illuminated in colours, is bound in deep brown calf, delicately ornamented with gold and blind tooling, and measures 8¼ by 5½ inches.

In the centre is a small royal coat of arms with a specially cut border, ensigned with a large royal crown and flanked by the initials M R. A broad rectangular fillet of gold and blind lines runs parallel with the edges of the boards, the gold being the inner of all, and mitred at the corners. This fillet marked by gold lines is ornamented along its length by impressions of a small arabesque cluster and a rosette, and at each of the outer corners is a large fleuron.

This binding is one of the most finely executed of any that can without doubt be attributed to Berthelet. The stamps used upon it are original in design, and although the Italian feeling is still evident, it is not so marked as in many other instances. The curious plan of adorning a fillet with impressions of small detached stamps is, I think, originally an Italian idea, but it is found more frequently on Berthelet's bindings than it is on those of any other master. Sometimes it occurs on fillets which are stained black, in which case a little bare place is left for the gold impression,—it is not gilded over the stain. Sometimes, as on this book, the fillet is left uncoloured. The unknown binder who worked for James I. and his sons used dots on fillets, but never stained them; and Samuel Mearne, royal binder to Charles II., revived the plan of gilding on a black fillet, but he did not carry it out to such an elaborate extent as did Berthelet, only using dots or dotted lines.

1554. Expositio Beati Ambrosii episcopi super apocalypsin. Lutetiae, 1554; measures 9¼ by 6½ inches, and is bound by Berthelet in dark brown calf, tooled in gold, with a few blind lines. In the centre is an ornamental cartouche enclosed within a rectangular border, and bearing the royal coat of arms of Queen Mary, crowned, and flanked by two scrolls; this is enclosed by a circle of wavy flames, and again by an outer irregularly shaped border of curves, straight lines, and arabesques. The space between the flamed circle and the outer arabesque line is filled with a powdering of small circular stamps.

The rectangular outer border is composed of straight lines in gold and blind, with centre fillet of an ornamental circular stamp crossed with arabesques of Italian character. The inner corners of the rectangle are filled with a trefoil stamp and the outer corners with an ornamental fleuron. There are the remains of two green silk ties on the front edge of each of the boards. The book is not in a good condition, the back having been entirely spoiled and tooled with recent stamps.

1555. Epitome omnium operum divi Aurelii Augustini, etc. Coloniae, 1549; measures 12½ by 8¼ inches, and is bound in brown calf, tooled in gold, with some blind lines. In the centre is the royal coat of arms of Queen Mary, crowned, and flanked by two arabesque curves, contained within a circle stained black, with waved rays of gold issuing outwards. The coat is enclosed by a long upright rectangular fillet stained black, interlaced by another in diamond shape of similar width, also stained black. The spaces within these two fillets are filled with gold curves and arabesques, except the two small triangles flanking the centre, which have the initials M R.

The black fillets are enclosed by a double border; the inner one, broken in four places by the points of the diamond, is thickly ornamented with corner fleurons and arabesque scrolls, the outer closely filled with a handsome arabesque made with two reversed curves. Outside all is another black rectangular fillet, with fleurons at the outer corners.

This is one of the finest calf bindings Berthelet made for Queen Mary, and it is wonderfully well preserved, the leather being only a little discoloured and the gold bright and clear. The black on the fillets is also in good condition.

1555. Bonner. A profitable and necessarye doctrine. London (1555); is bound in pale brown calf for Queen Mary, and tooled in gold, without any black in the fillets. In the centre is the royal coat of arms flanked by two scrolls and enclosed within a flanked circle. This circle is contained in a diamond-shaped fillet, with leaf stamps in the upper and lower corners, beyond which is a rectangular border of Italian fashion, made by small circles intersected by arabesques,—a favourite pattern of Berthelet's, and very effective. The four inner corners of the parallelogram are filled with arabesque ornaments, and the outer corners have small fleurons. All the stamps are well known.